THE MODERN GIRL'S BO
TORTURE!

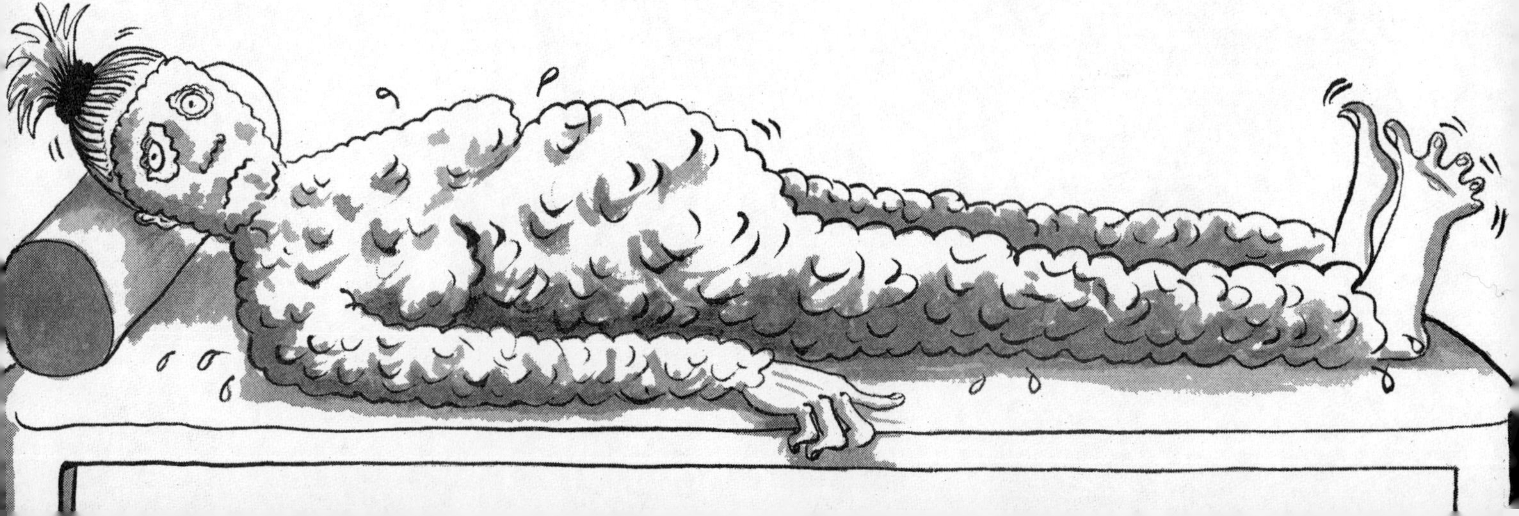

Alison Everitt has also written:
The Condom Book for Girls; *That's Fashion!*; and *Revenge of the Essex Girls* with Cathy Hopkins (Robsons).

An OPTIMA Book

First published in 1992 by Optima

A CIP catalogue record for this book
is available from the British Library.

ISBN 0 356 20971 7

Printed and bound in Great Britain by
The Guernsey Press Co. Ltd.,
Guernsey, Channel Islands.

Optima
A Division of
Little, Brown & Company (UK) Limited
165 Great Dover Street
London SE1 4YA

Dedicated to women everywhere who, in the constant battle with their bodies, have been on one diet or another for most of their lives; who have tried to be Jane Fonda but failed miserably ... and to those who stare longingly at scalpels...

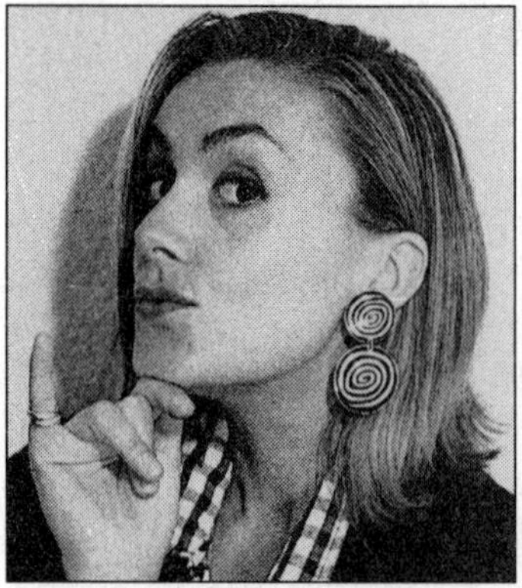

**ALISON EVERITT.
AUTHOR.**

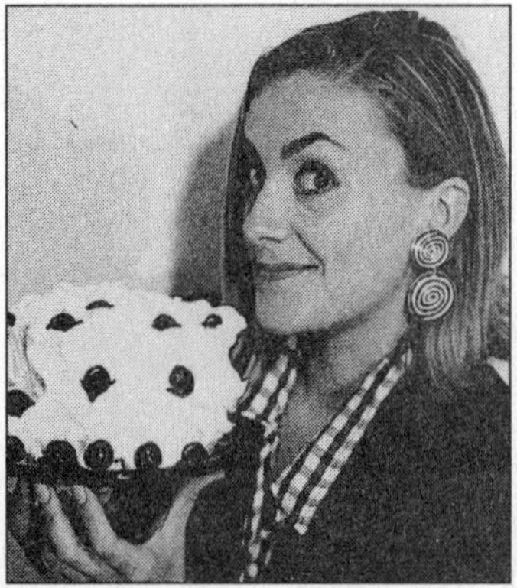

Lover of fine foods...

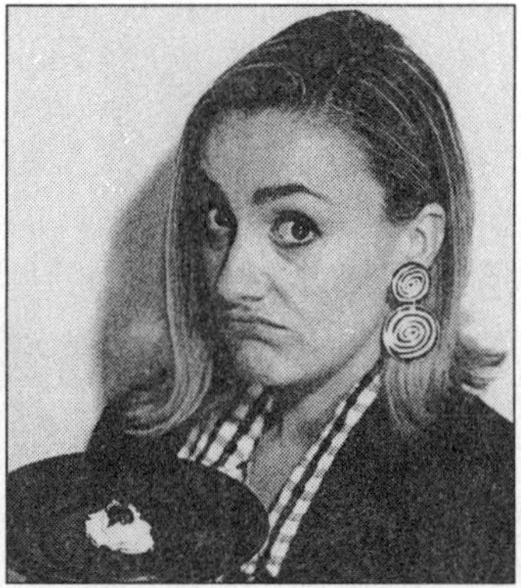

Diet Attempter...

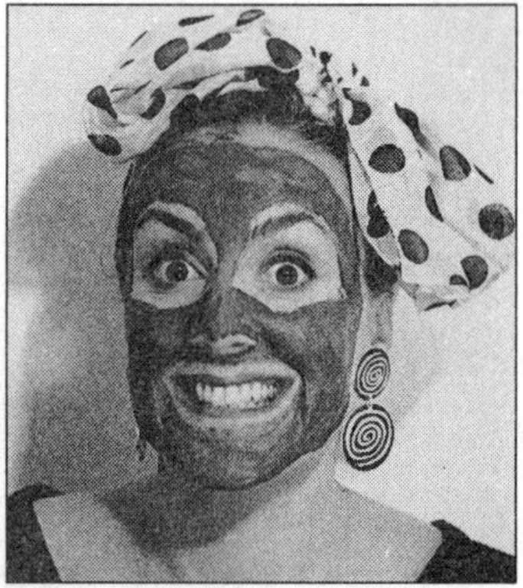

Face Pack Applier...

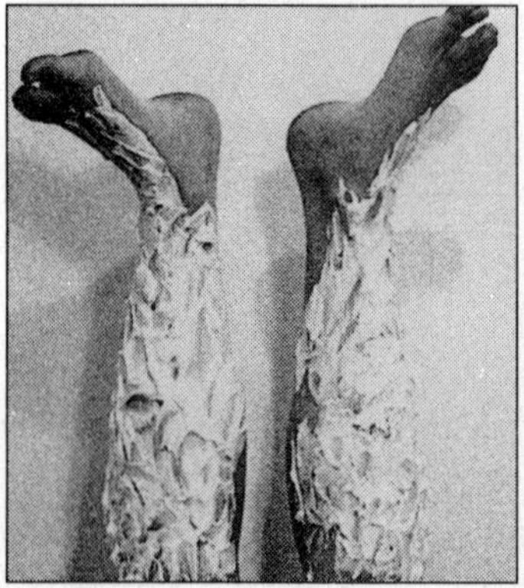

Hair Remover...

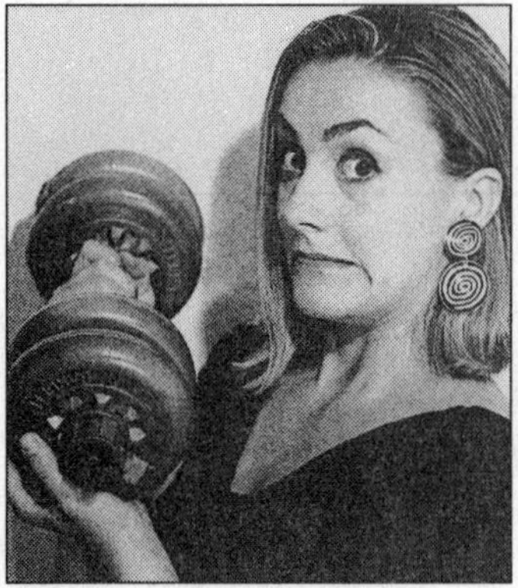

Exerciser...

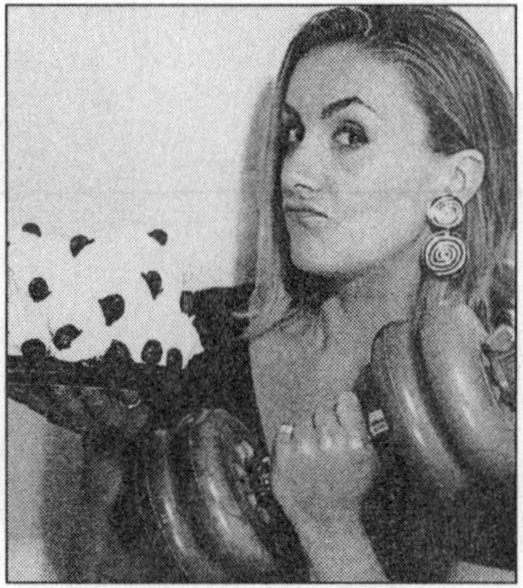

...Exerciser!...

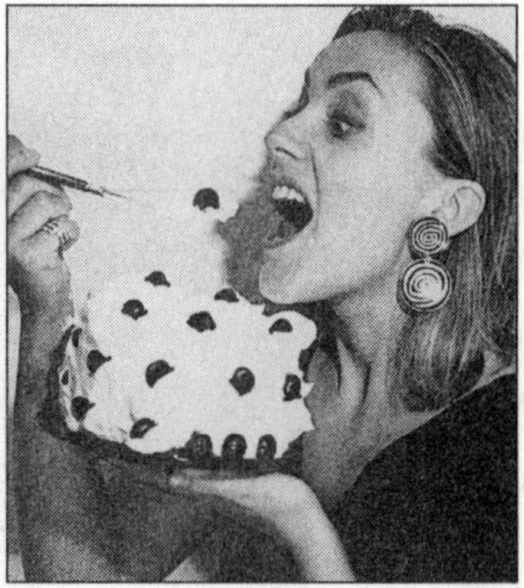

...Oh well....

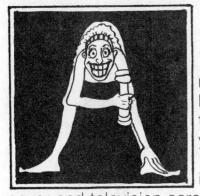

re you Perfect Woman? Do you exercise every day? Have you got lithe, firm thighs and a stomach you can throw rocks at? When you walk, does nothing move but your feet? Do you never, *never* suffer from PMT?

... Didn't think so. Perfect Woman is very hard to find in real life, yet there she is on every poster, magazine cover and television screen, telling us how we should be feeling, what we should be wearing, and which size we ought to be. This is where the TORTURE starts. We torture ourselves for giving into pressure and starving ourselves. We torture ourselves for eating one Danish Pastry in rebellion ... and then we torture ourselves for torturing ourselves.

But if we face the fact that most women mess up their make-up, make a hash of their hair, worry about their womb and are fed up with feeling fat, then life doesn't seem half as bad! So, read on...

HEALTH

VITAMIN B
H-R-T
ROYAL JELLY
WATER RETENTION TABLETS
ASPIRIN

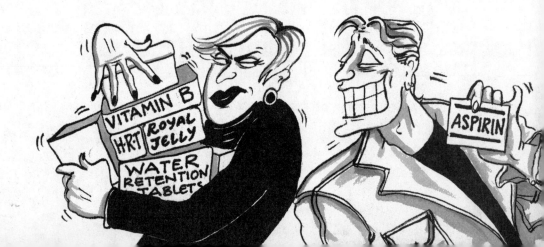

Men only have a couple of extra body parts to us. We're positively *riddled* with spare bits and pieces that can suddenly collapse. We've come to realise that unless we want to spend the rest of our lives in bed we have to pull ourselves together and get on with it. (With the loving support of our *men* of course!)

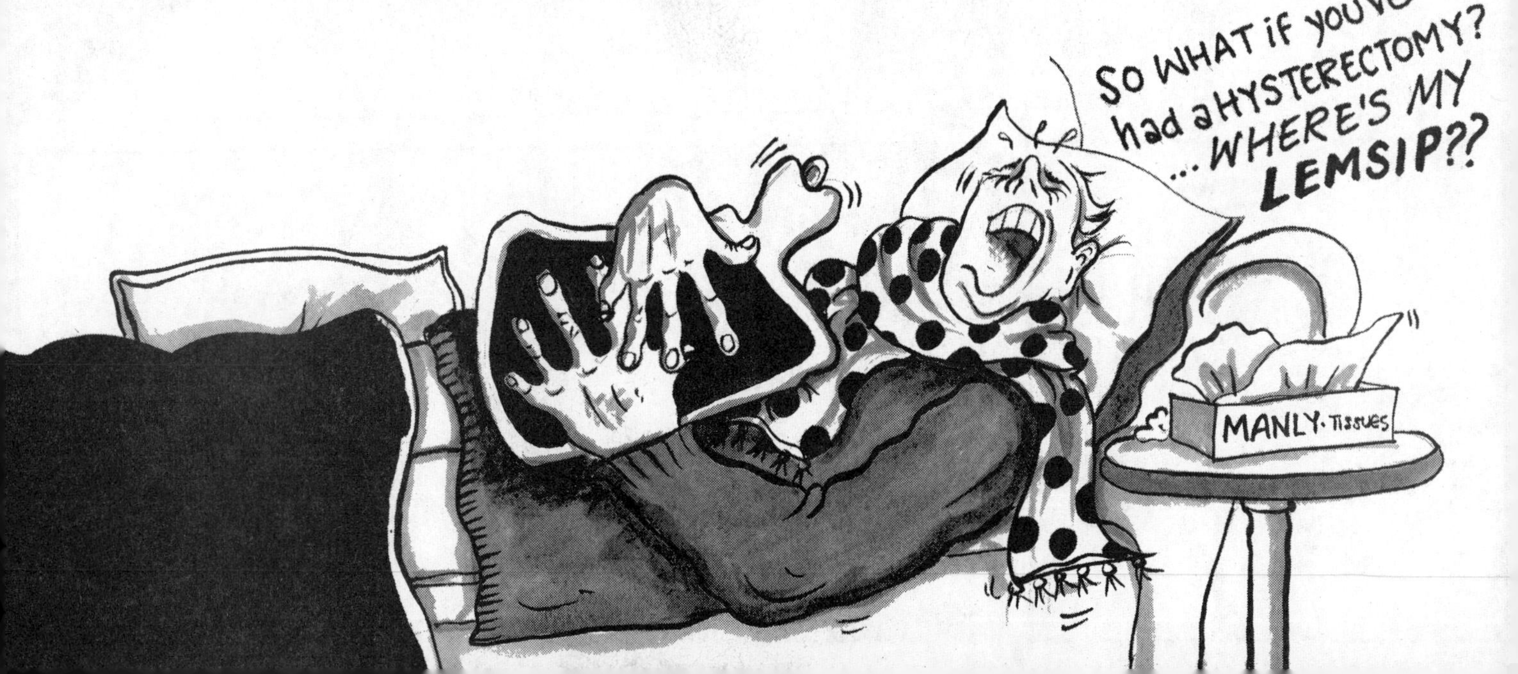
SO WHAT if you've had a HYSTERECTOMY? ...WHERE'S MY LEMSIP??
MANLY. Tissues

Despite our sturdy survival attitude concerning our bodies, we turn into gibbering wrecks when it comes to the DENTIST...

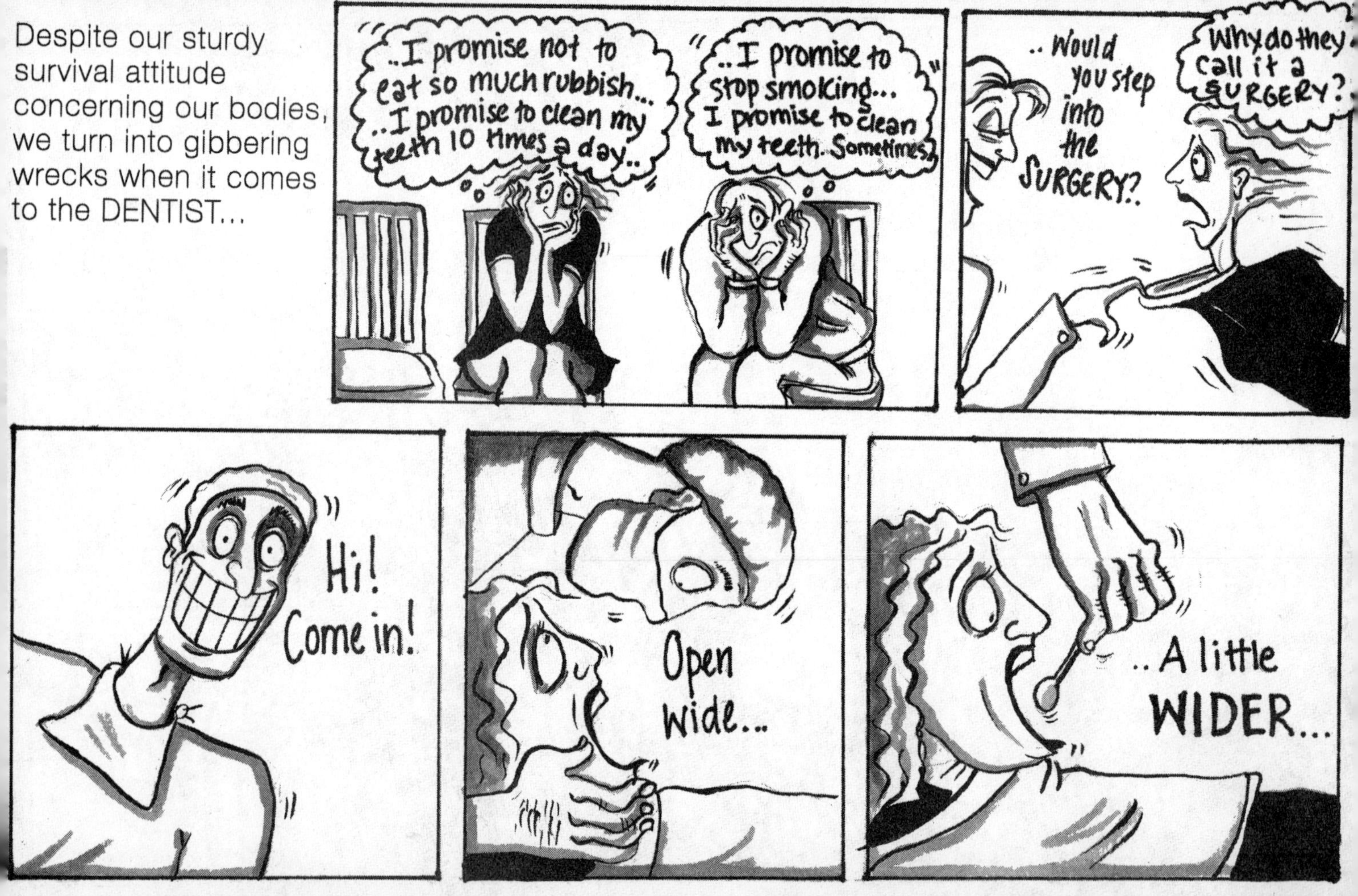
..I promise not to eat so much rubbish... ..I promise to clean my teeth 10 times a day..
..I promise to stop smoking... I promise to clean my teeth. Sometimes?
.. Would you step into the SURGERY?.
Why do they call it a SURGERY?
Hi! Come in!
Open wide...
.. A little WIDER...

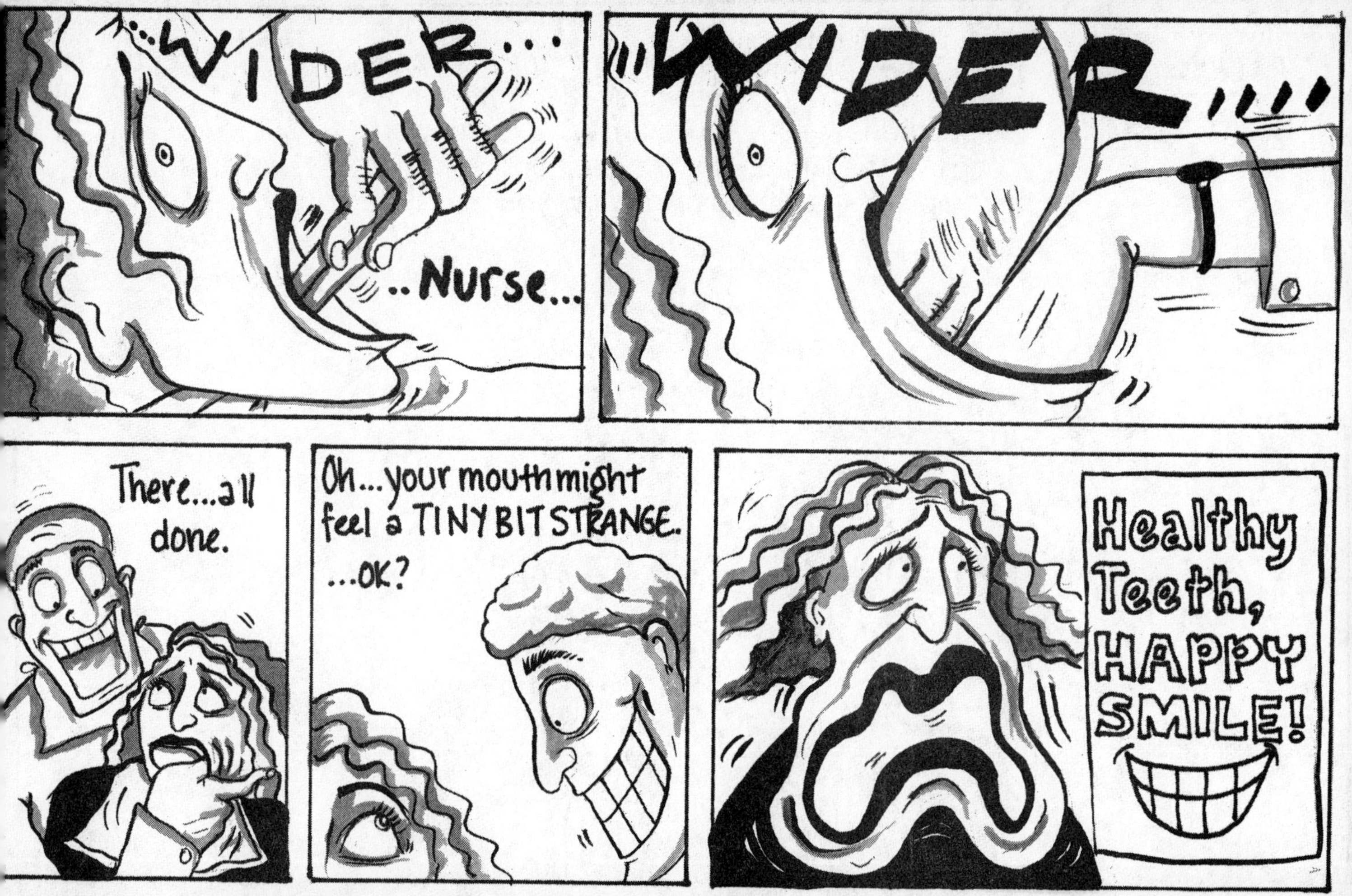
...WIDER...
..Nurse...
"WIDER!!!!!
There...all done.
Oh...your mouth might feel a TINY BIT STRANGE.
...OK?
Healthy Teeth, HAPPY SMILE!

WAITING ROOMS:

After a few minutes in a waiting room you can easily end up feeling ten times worse than when you went in. Forget the fact that they're always too stuffy and full of people with germs… *nothing* can top the feeling of waiting for a complete stranger to re-arrange your private parts.

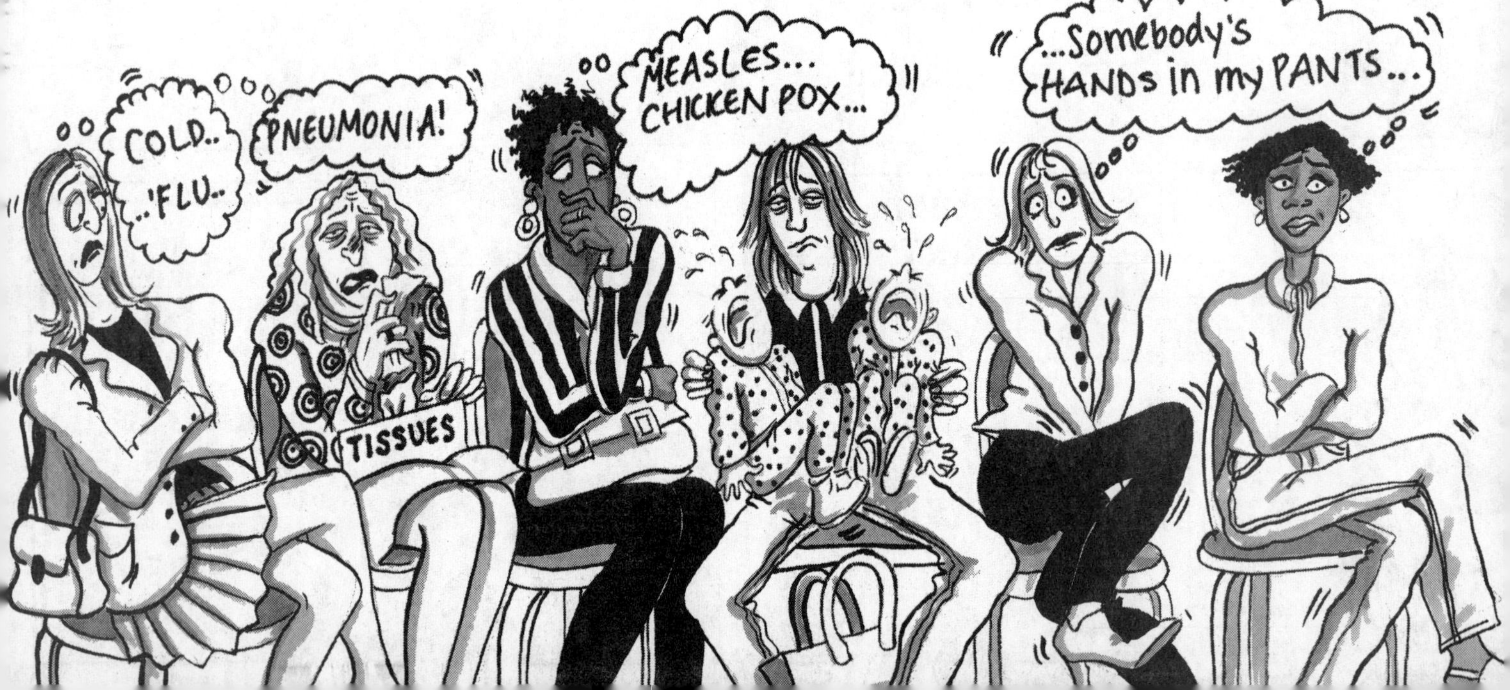

COLD.. ..'FLU..
PNEUMONIA!
MEASLES… CHICKEN POX…
…Somebody's HANDS in my PANTS…
TISSUES

... and if THAT wasn't enough to send you rushing for an oxygen tent, you find you're not even allowed any simple distractions...

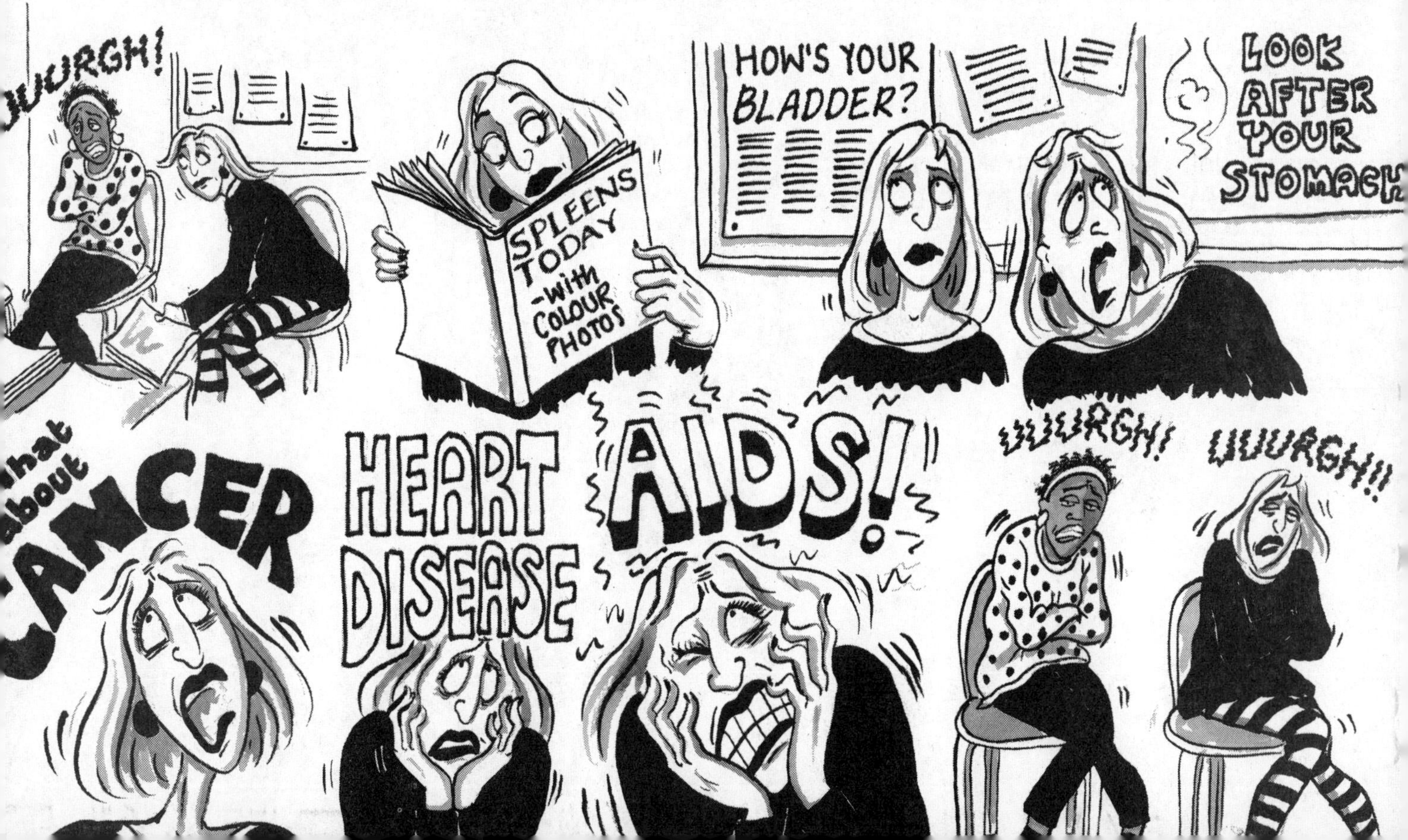
UUURGH!
SPLEENS TODAY -with COLOUR PHOTOS
HOW'S YOUR BLADDER?
LOOK AFTER YOUR STOMACH
what about CANCER
HEART DISEASE
AIDS!
UUURGH!
UUURGH!!

DOCTORS ...

Nothing is more important than finding a good doctor, because if something should suddenly go wrong, we don't want to be attended to by someone who is likely to make us WORSE. Unfortunately we have to find a doctor that we like, can trust, who doesn't treat us like an imbecile, *and* who has a surgery within a certain distance from our house. So most of the time we have to put up with what we can GET.

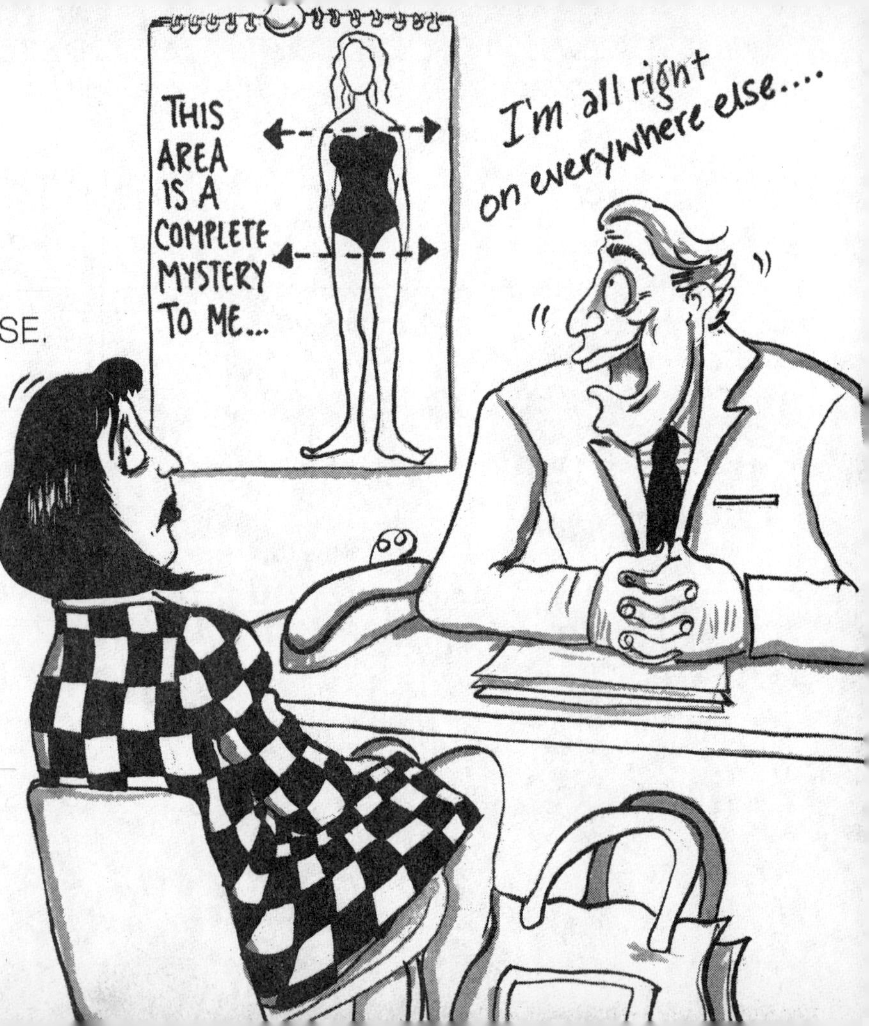
THIS AREA IS A COMPLETE MYSTERY TO ME...
I'm all right on everywhere else....

It's not surprising that some of us try alternative methods ... but they aren't exactly perfect either. If you decide to diagnose yourself from medical books ...

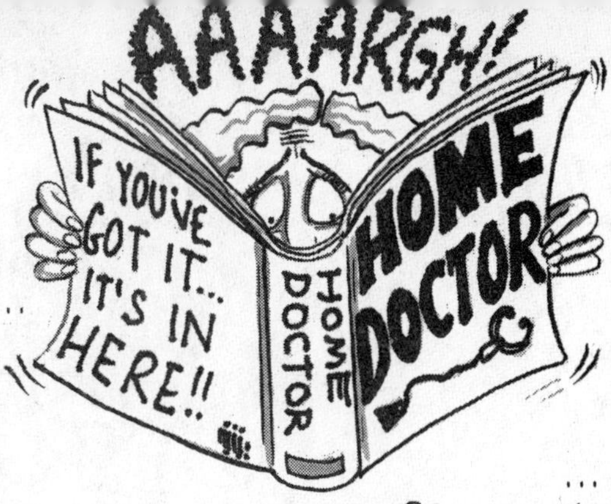
AAAARGH!
IF YOU'VE GOT IT... IT'S IN HERE!!
HOME DOCTOR
HOME DOCTOR

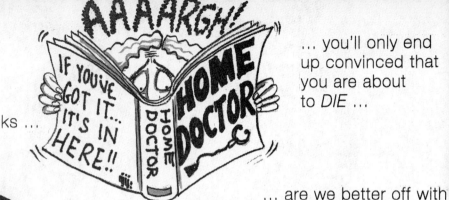

... you'll only end up convinced that you are about to *DIE* ...

... Homeopathic treatments are often linked with pasty-faced vegans in unfortunate knitwear who look worse than we do ...

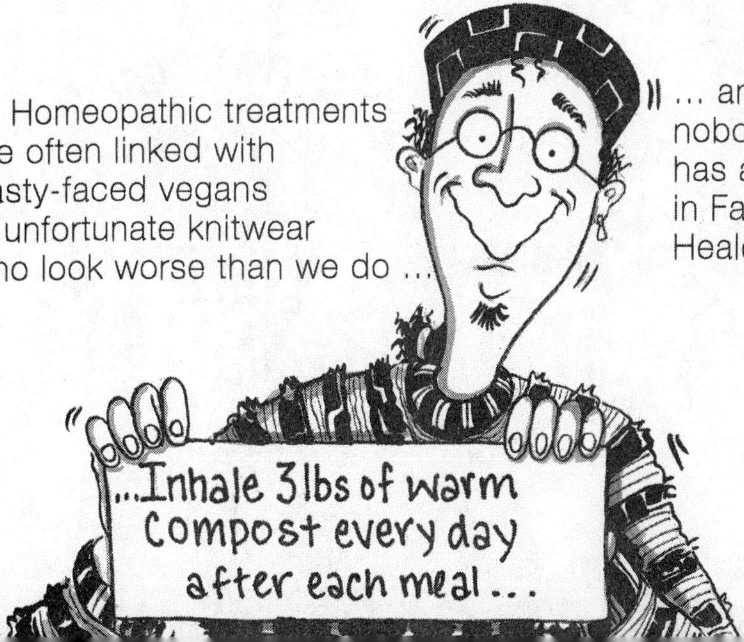
...Inhale 3lbs of warm Compost every day after each meal...

... and as nobody really has any faith in Faith Healers ...

... are we better off with the traditional GP?

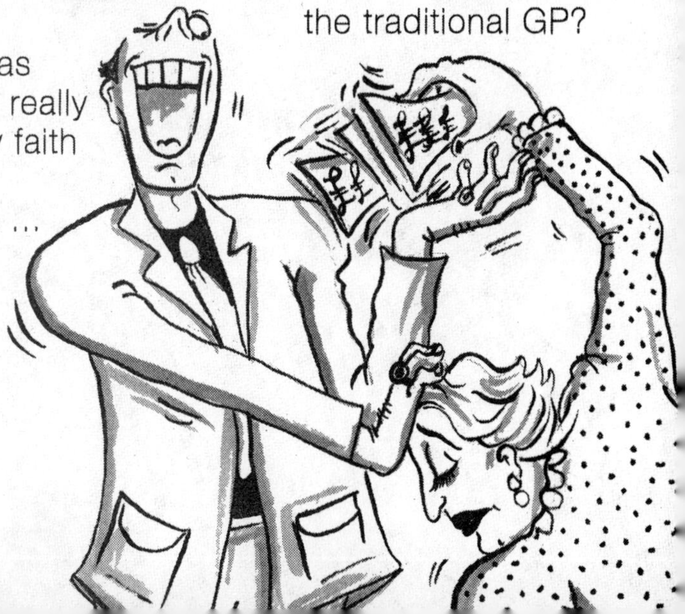

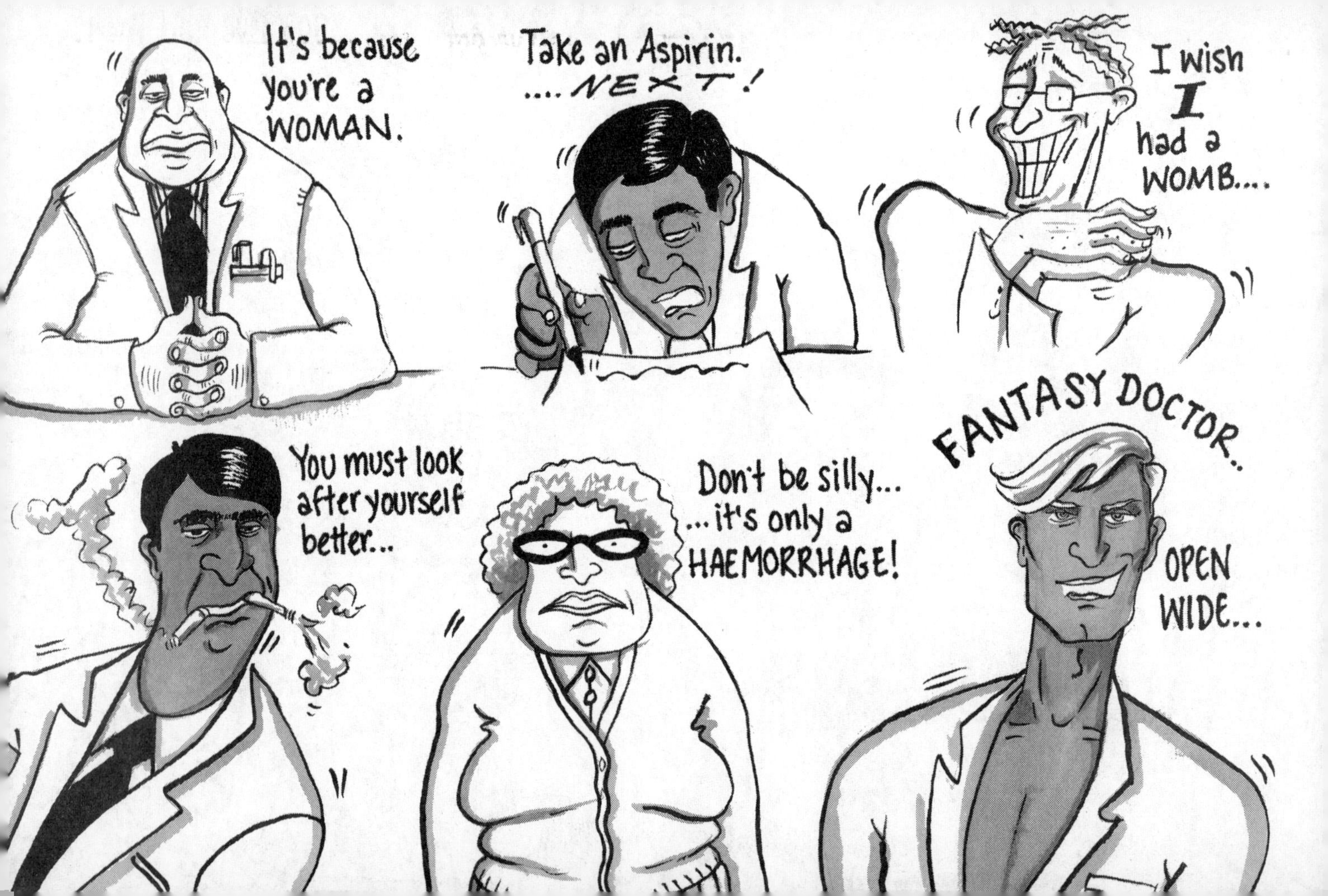
It's because you're a WOMAN.
Take an Aspirin. .... NEXT!
I wish I had a WOMB....
You must look after yourself better...
Don't be silly... ...it's only a HAEMORRHAGE!
FANTASY DOCTOR..
OPEN WIDE...

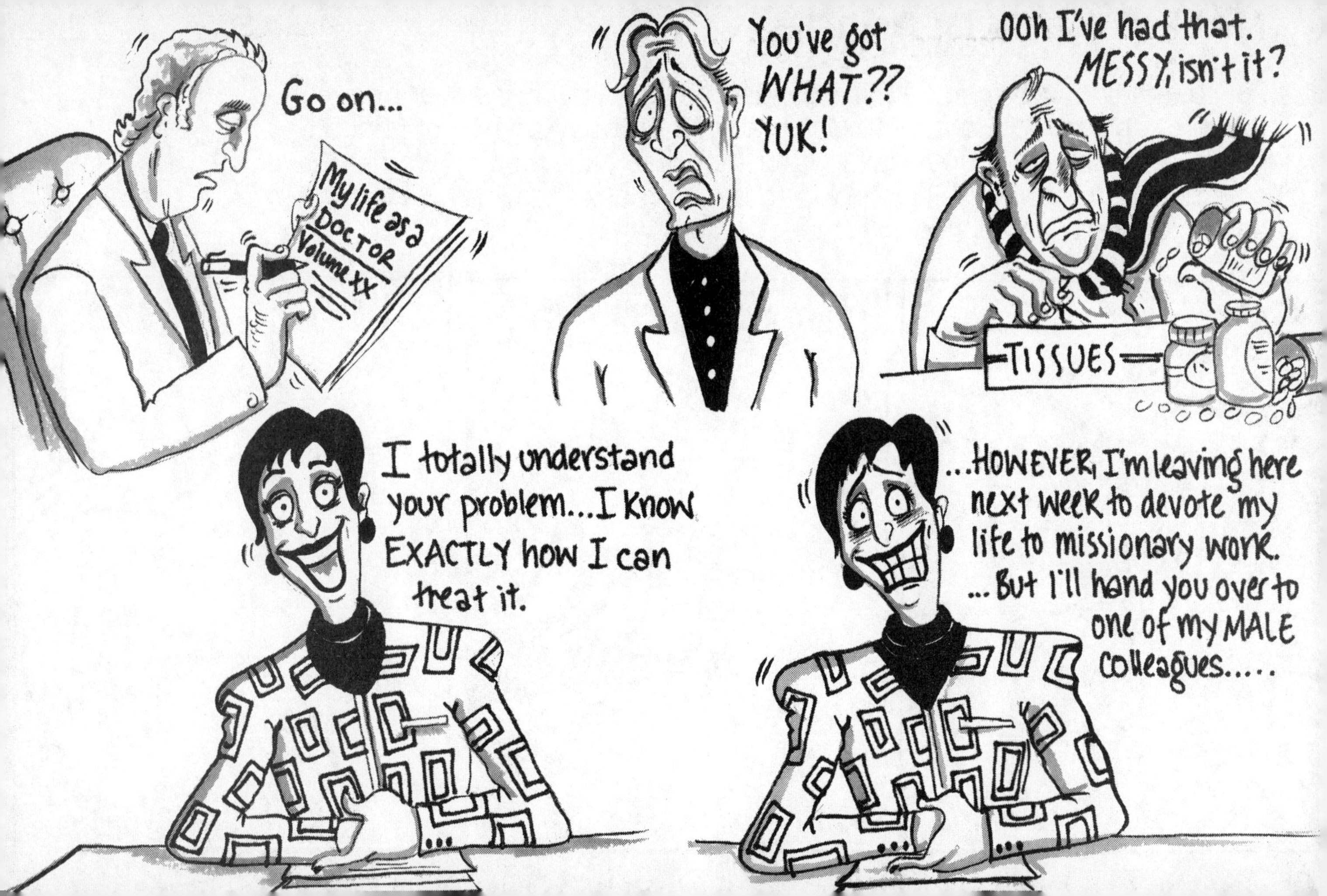

Go on...
My life as a DOCTOR Volume XX
You've got WHAT?? YUK!
OOh I've had that. MESSY, isn't it?
TISSUES
I totally understand your problem...I know EXACTLY how I can treat it.
...HOWEVER, I'm leaving here next week to devote my life to missionary work. ...But I'll hand you over to one of my MALE colleagues.....

MALE GYNAECOLOGISTS

I can't imagine why men become gynaecologists. It would never occur to me to spend most of my life giving advice on body parts that I hadn't got ... and they can't possibly do it for the view. I know some women have confidence in them, but if *I'm* going to be internally examined, I want to have it done by someone who at least knows what it FEELS LIKE!

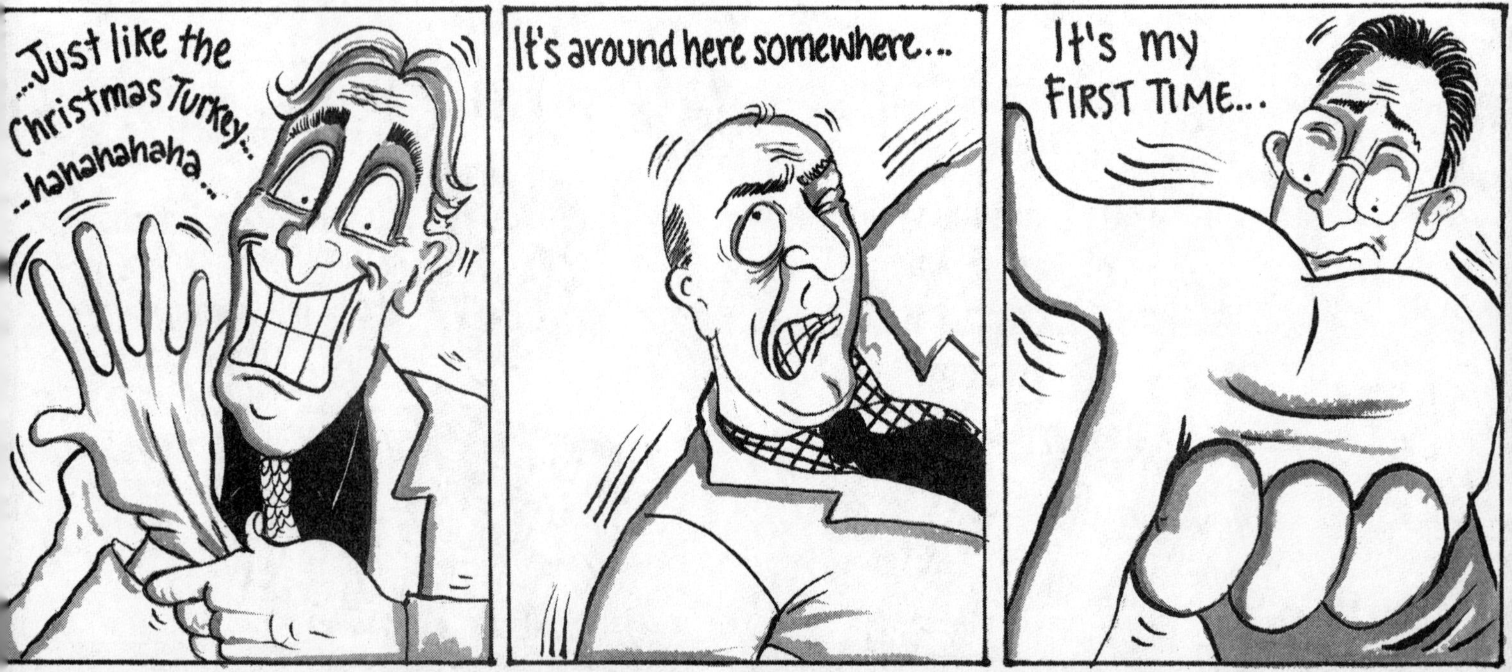
...Just like the Christmas Turkey... ...hahahahaha...
It's around here somewhere...
It's my FIRST TIME...

SMEAR TESTS:

A crucial part of women's health, but hindered by the fact that it involves the removal of your knickers. This puts an awful lot of women off, especially if your doctor invites a group of students to watch, or thinks it's funny to ask if the earth moved for you.

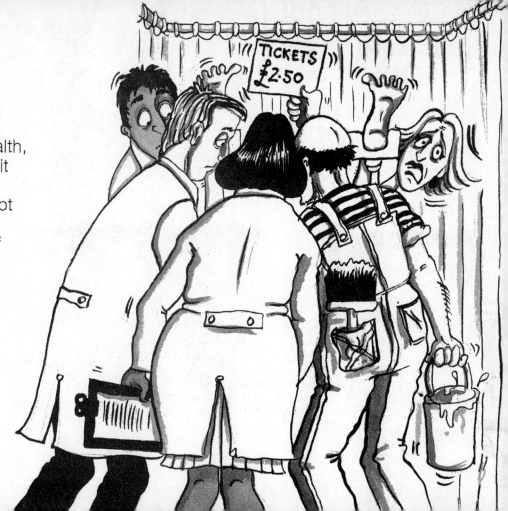

PRE-MENSTRUAL TENSION ...

Smirking men call it "That Time Of The Month," close friends call it DANGER TIME; you have a bloated stomach, swollen, aching boobs, manky hair and a short temper.

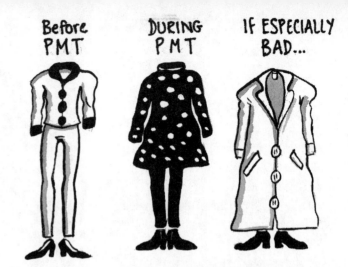

Before PMT

DURING PMT

IF ESPECIALLY BAD...

If you're anything like me you also trip over paving slabs, drop your shopping, mess up your work and try to cope with life when you feel like death ...

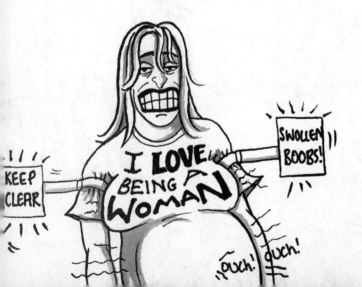

KEEP CLEAR

SWOLLEN BOOBS!

I LOVE BEING A WOMAN

"ouch! ouch!

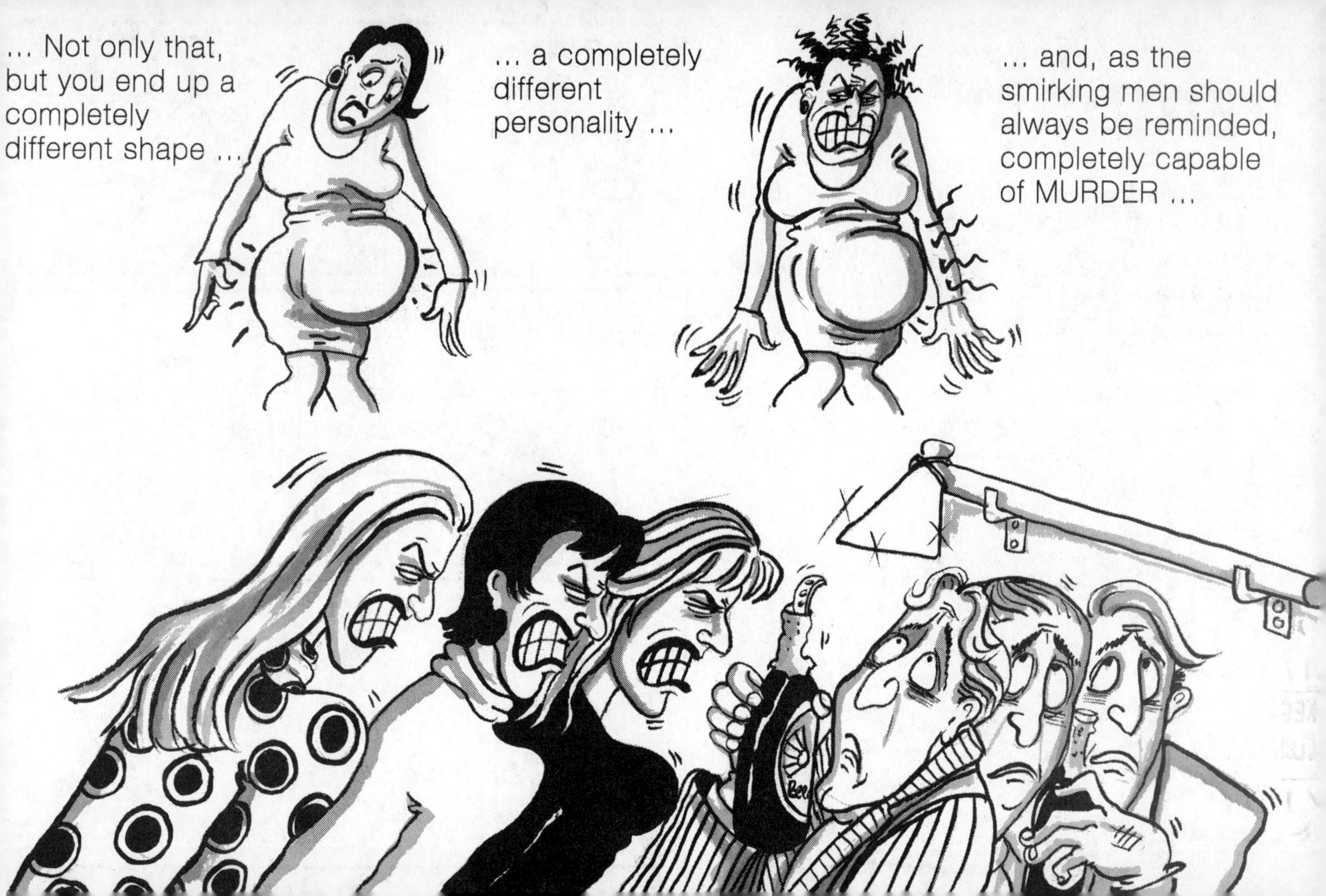
... Not only that, but you end up a completely different shape ...
... a completely different personality ...
... and, as the smirking men should always be reminded, completely capable of MURDER ...

PERIODS!

Years ago, periods were a secret, feminine mystery that should be silently endured and never, *never* discussed in public. In old movies, women never had periods, were practically never seen when pregnant, and always gave birth behind closed doors. If you believed the adverts we still have on TV, you'd think that nothing had changed.

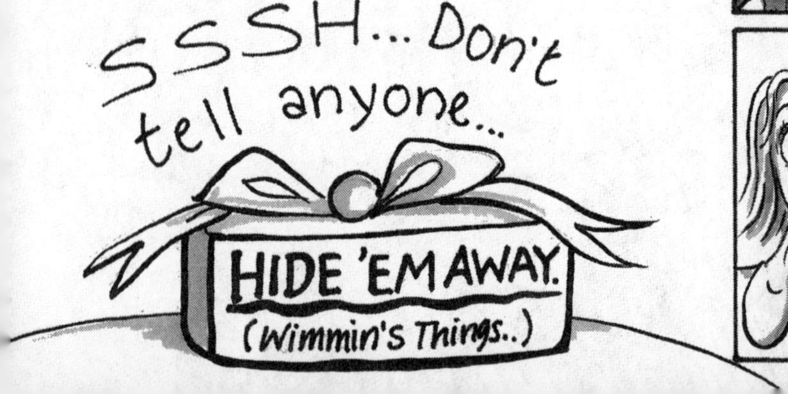

SSSH... Don't tell anyone...
HIDE 'EM AWAY.
(Wimmin's Things..)

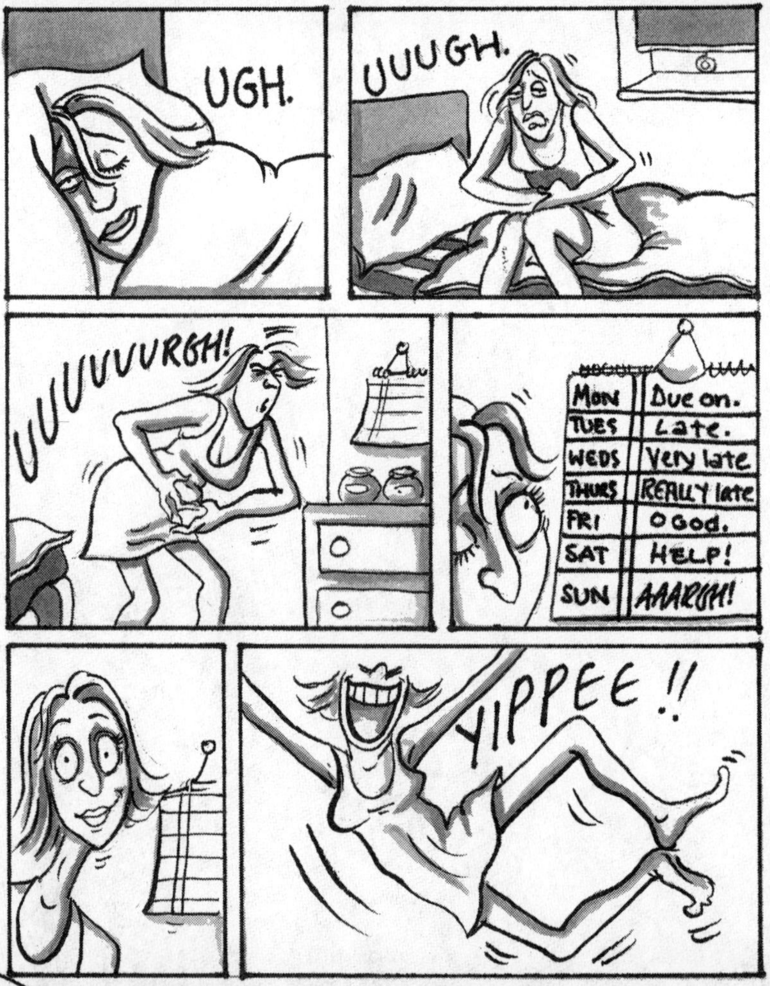

UGH.
UUUGH.
UUUUUUURGH!
MON Due on.
TUES Late.
WEDS Very late
THURS REALLY late
FRI O God.
SAT HELP!
SUN AAARGH!
YIPPEE!!

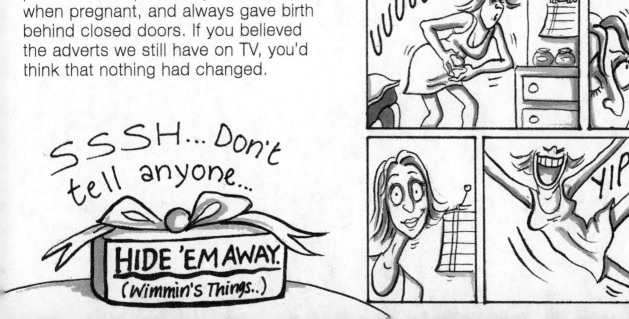

It's no wonder we don't exactly look forward to our periods, when we're surrounded by older women spending most of their lives rolling around the floor in agony.

UUUURGH...
AROMATHERAPY
MEGA EVENING PRIMROSE OIL

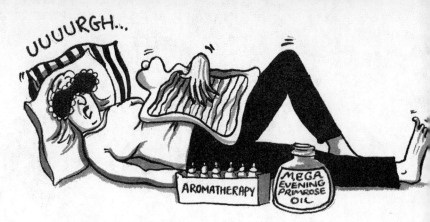

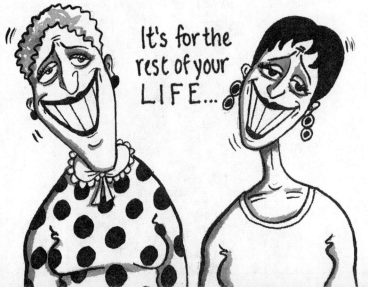

It's for the rest of your LIFE...

Either that, or they're telling gruesome tales from their past using encouraging phrases like The Curse or The Red Plague. If that wasn't bad enough, when we start our first one they hover about with a "Join the Club" look on their face. I say bring back the old movies!

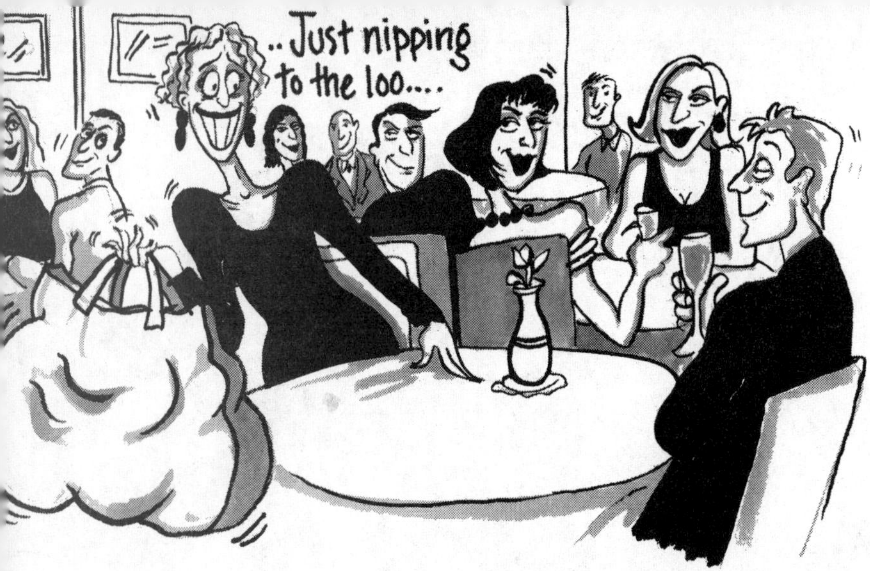
..Just nipping to the loo....

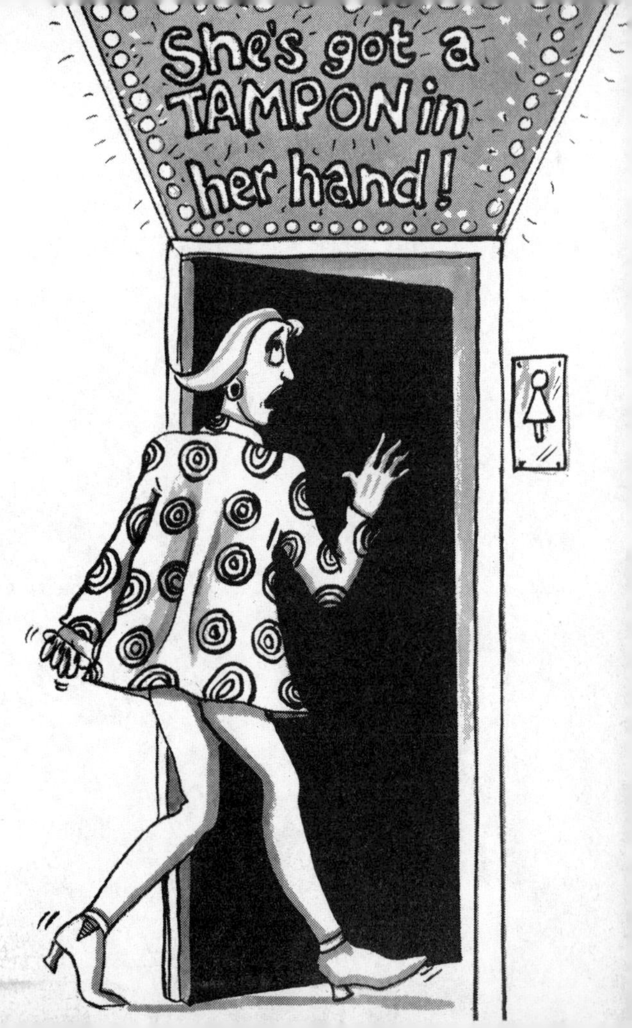
She's got a TAMPON in her hand!

An obvious sign that a period was going on used to be when someone took a handbag with them wherever they went. Nowadays sanitary goods are made so compact that they're easier to carry about and, if it bothers you, no-one can know what you're doing.

The only perk that comes with periods is when we talk about them as often and as loudly as we can, especially in male company, and see how long it takes to make them squirm, turn green and eventually beg for a window open.

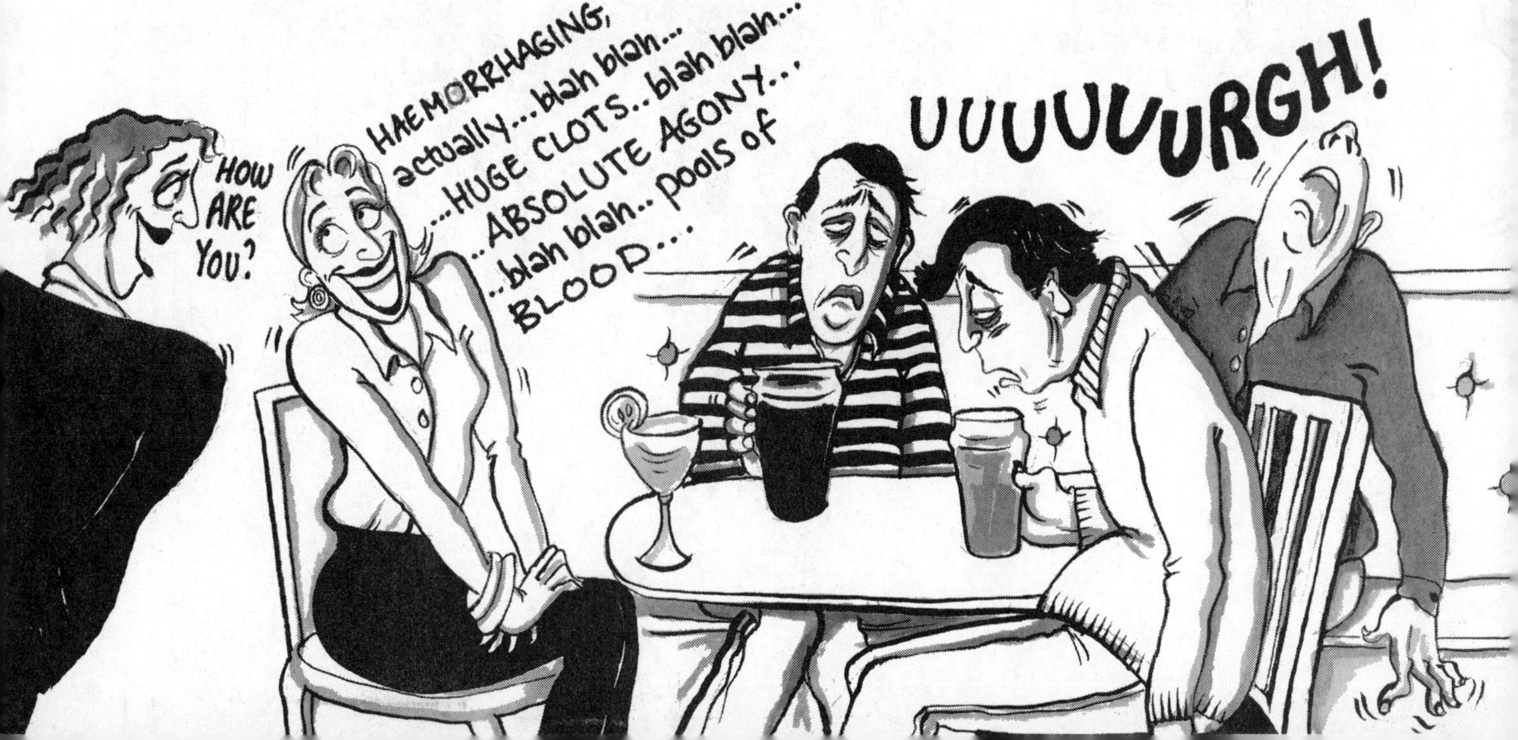
HOW ARE YOU?
HAEMORRHAGING, actually...blah blah... ...HUGE CLOTS...blah blah... ...ABSOLUTE AGONY... ..blah blah.. pools of BLOOD....
UUUUUURGH!

If men had periods we'd never hear the last of it. Family celebrations would break out when the first one arrived, Bank Holidays would be declared in honour of Fertility ...

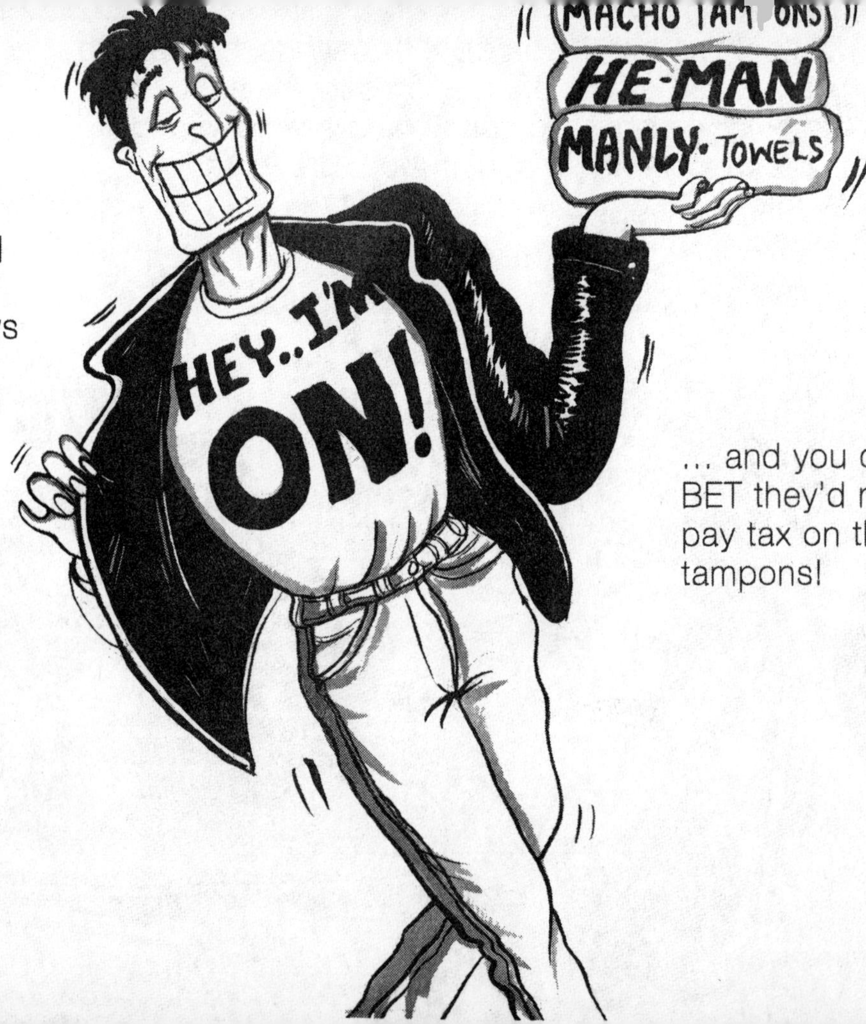
MACHO TAM ONS
HE-MAN
MANLY· TOWELS
HEY.. I'M
ON!

... and you can BET they'd never pay tax on their tampons!

And when it came to BUSINESS the country would grind to a complete halt as they took to their beds for the week.

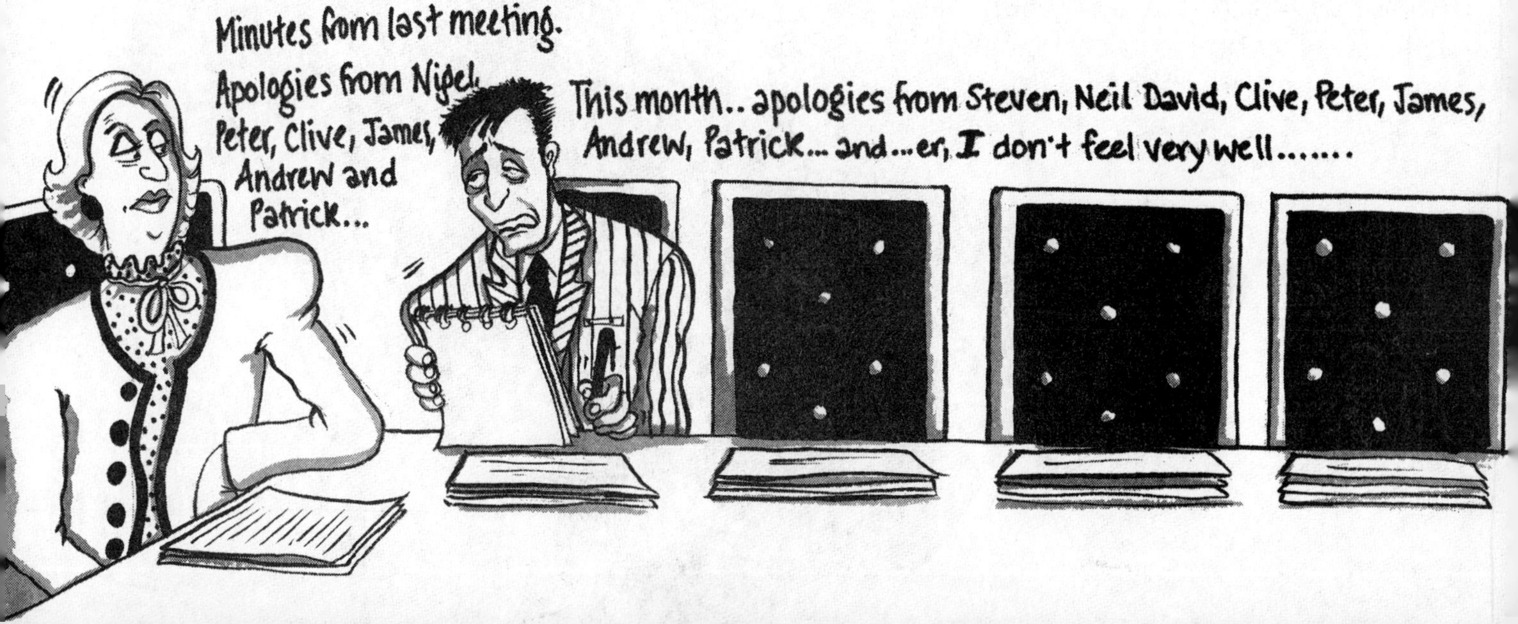
Minutes from last meeting.
Apologies from Nigel, Peter, Clive, James, Andrew and Patrick...
This month.. apologies from Steven, Neil David, Clive, Peter, James, Andrew, Patrick... and...er, I don't feel very well.......

Eventually the day will arrive when you'll have your last ever period. Unfortunately this means you're experiencing your MENOPAUSE. These days you have a choice whether you hang onto your periods and replace your hormones, or follow your course and get Hot Flushes. Either way you can end up hairy, absent-minded, shoplifting, and being attracted to skinny, spotty TOY BOYS. Something to look forward to, eh?

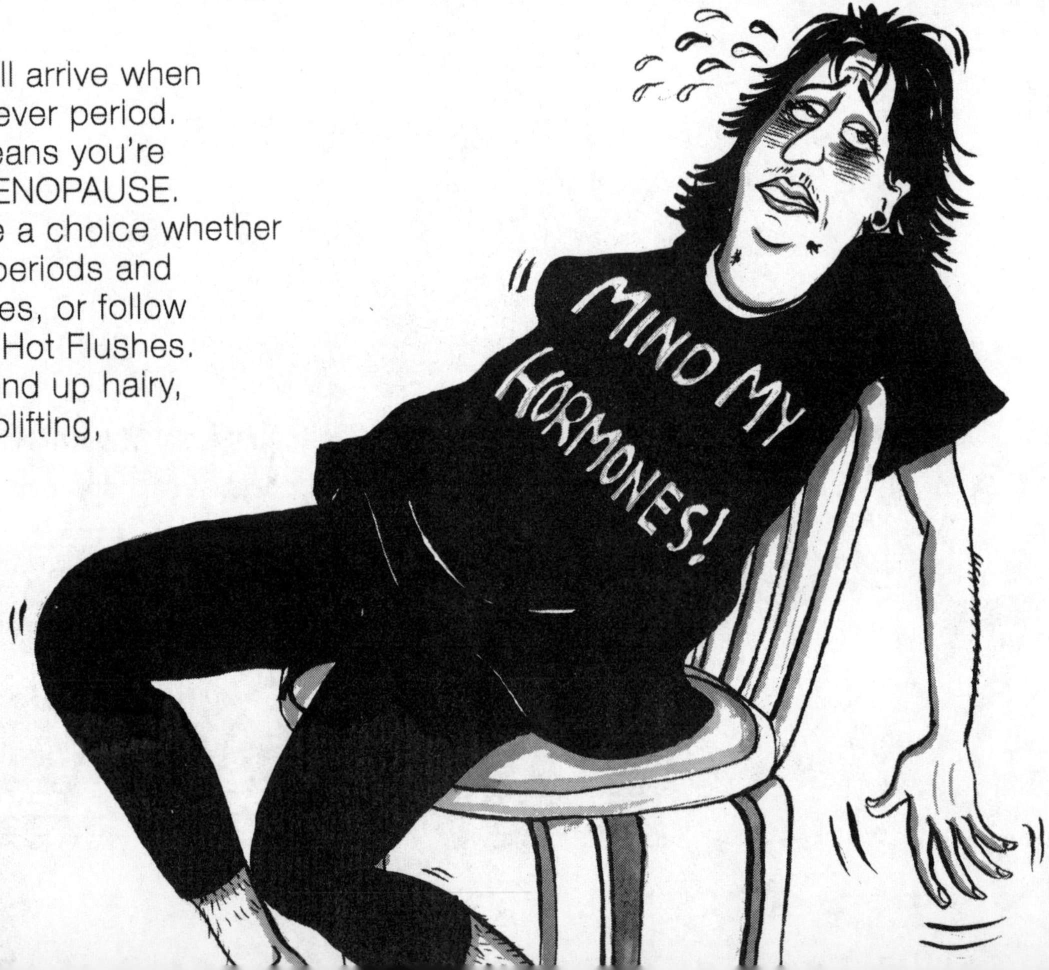
MIND MY HORMONES!

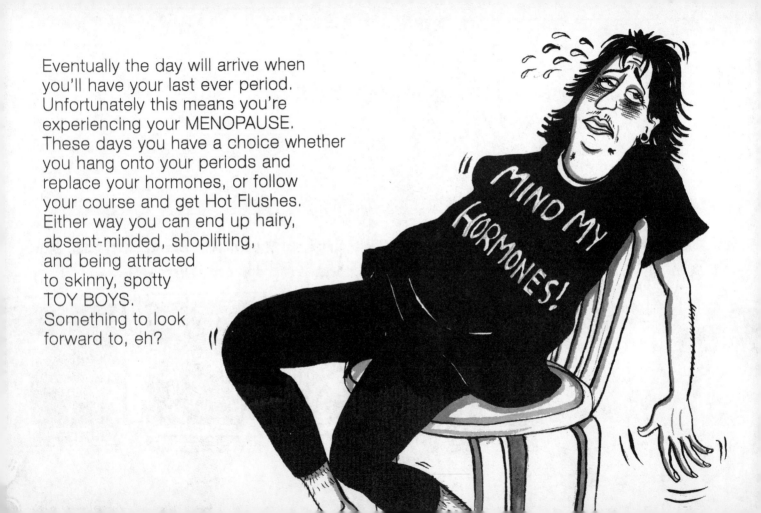

BEAUTY

GIVE UP!

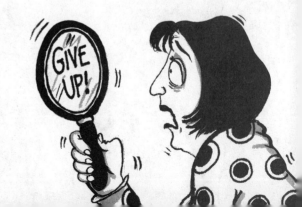

Keeping yourself attractive is a pressure that lies heavier on women than on men. The fantasy is that men grow more desirable as they grow more creased, whereas we are neglected and divorced if we don't smooth every wrinkle and whittle away every inch. The truth is that an awful lot of men should never be allowed out in daylight ... but the fantasy lives on and the Beauty Business thrives.

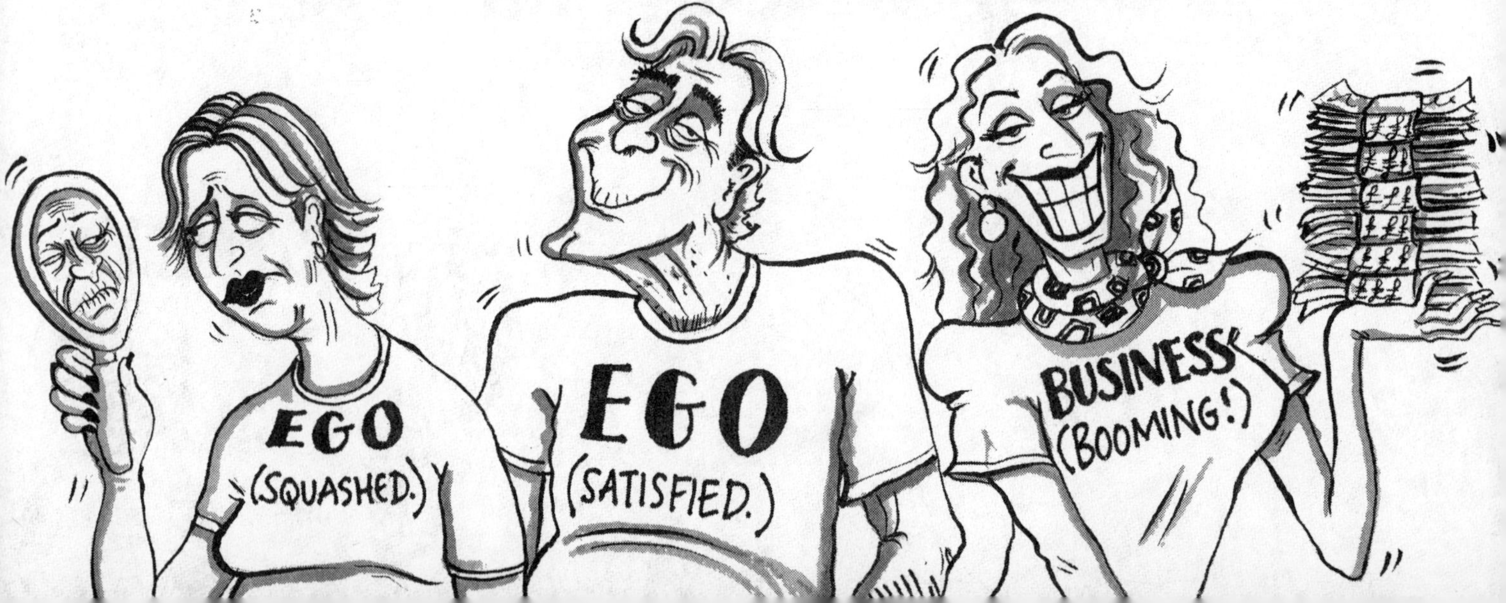
EGO
(SQUASHED.)
EGO
(SATISFIED.)
BUSINESS
(BOOMING!)

A large part of the Big Fat Fib, sorry, the Beauty Business, are the huge selection of creams, potions and lotions that promise a short cut to a long life of youth and beauty.

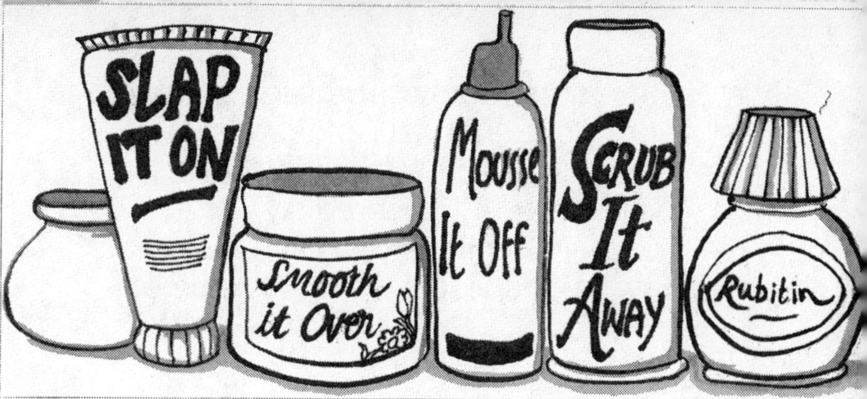
SLAP IT ON
Smooth it Over
Mousse It Off
Scrub It Away
Rubitin

They promise to wipe away wrinkles ...

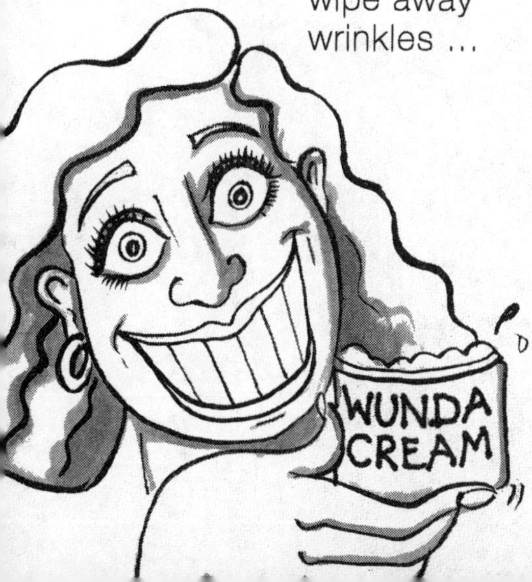
WUNDA CREAM

... slap away cellulite ...

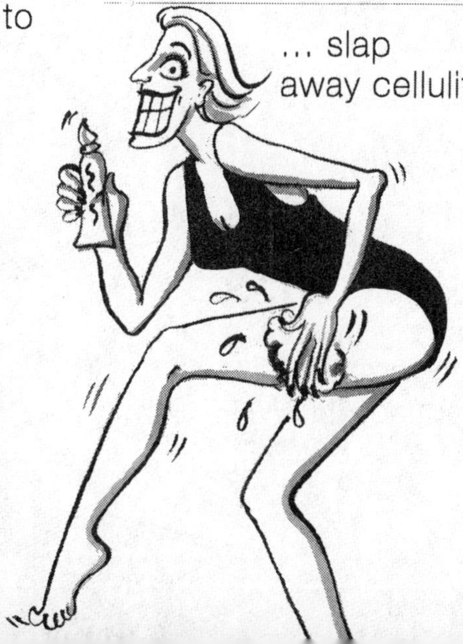

... and (if we didn't have a Trade Descriptions Act), to introduce you to the Man of your Dreams, make you a financial wizard, and lengthen your legs by at least ten inches.

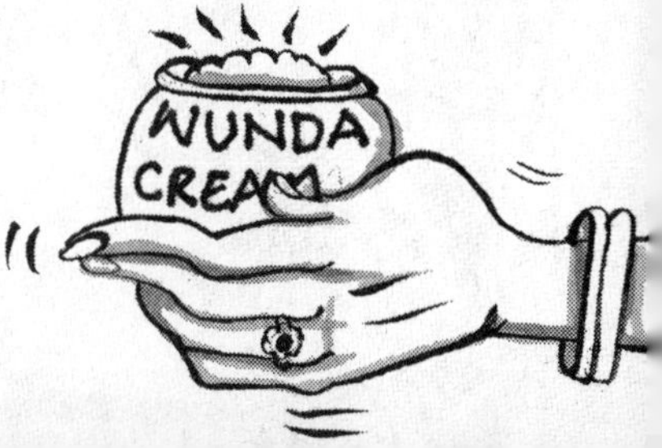
WUNDA CREAM

The latest attempts to combat ageing come in video form. Hour after hour of tape is dedicated to telling us how to oil, exfoliate, pamper and massage. It's incredibly hard, however, to do yourself, as you can't look in the mirror and at the video at the same time.

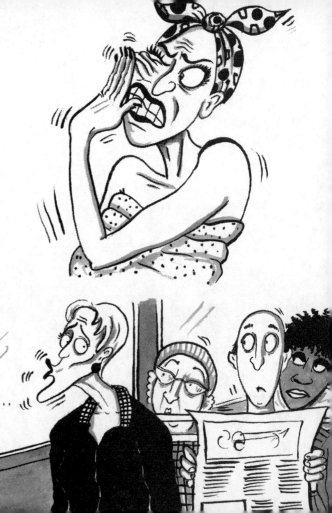

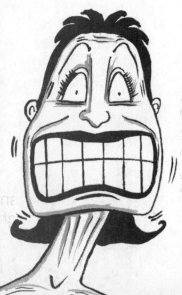

A new concept is FACERCISE, the pulling of extreme faces to stretch and tone muscles we don't usually use. According to the videos, you can practise ANYWHERE ...

And then there are people who produce videos that tell us how they manage to keep old age at bay.

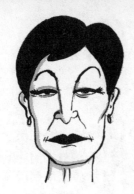

For example: this is Nancy. Nancy has never had plastic surgery ...

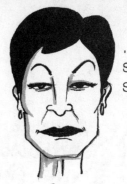

... and yet she looks so young!

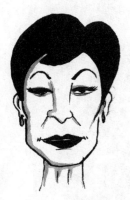

Nancy says you must work from the inside out. Nancy never eats fatty foods.

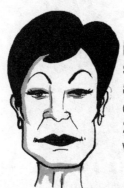

Nancy never stays out late, and never drinks less than 20 pints of water a day.

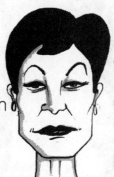

Nancy spends her time in front of the mirror being terrified of growing old. (Nancy also hasn't had a good laugh for 30 years.)

Most women don't go to the trouble of producing videos. If they've found a secret of eternal youth they'll happily tell anyone.

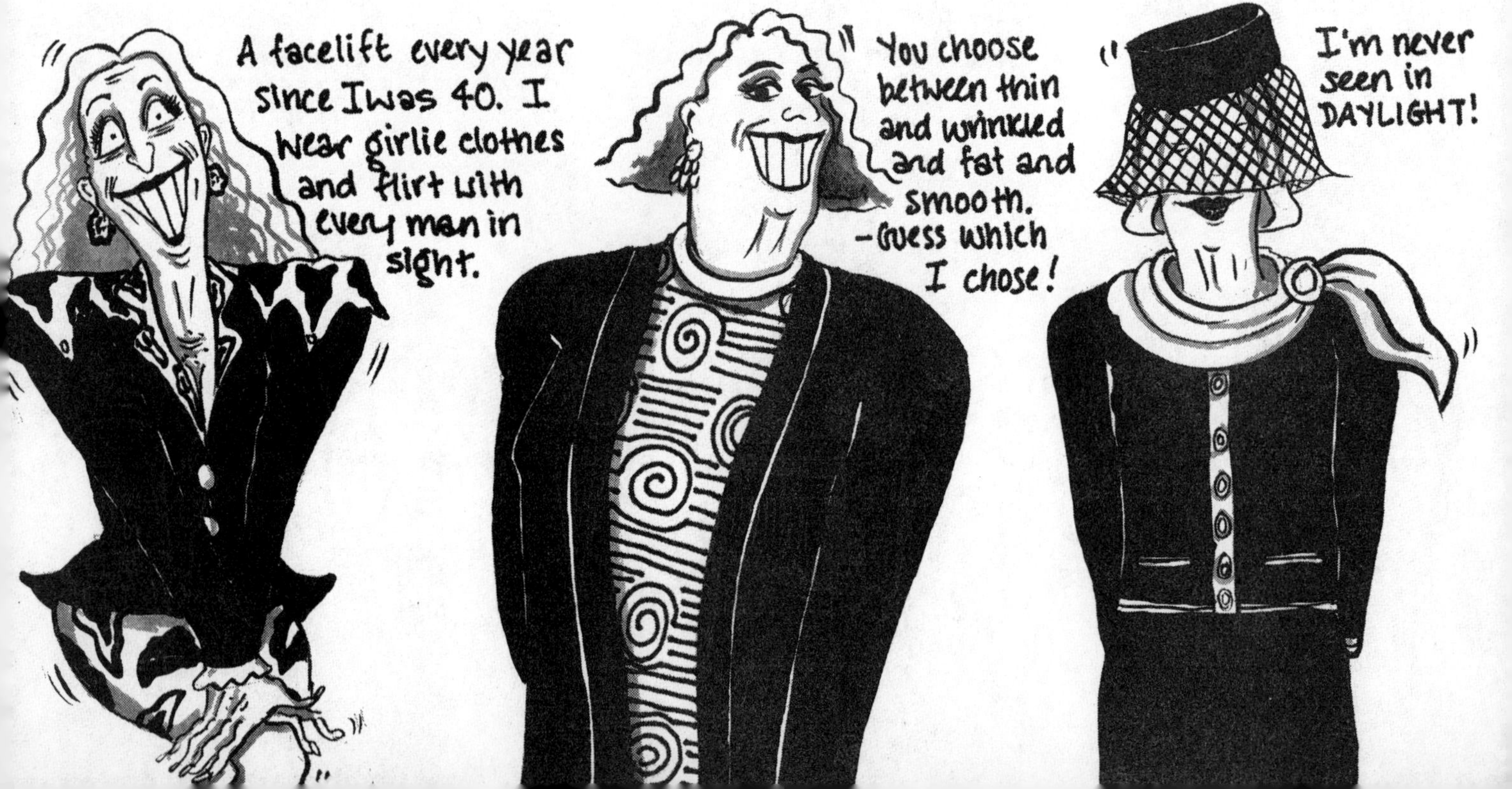
A facelift every year since I was 40. I wear girlie clothes and flirt with every man in sight.
You choose between thin and wrinkled and fat and smooth. - Guess which I chose!
I'm never seen in DAYLIGHT!

MAKE-UP ...

When we're teenagers, we won't leave the house without our make-up on. As a result we get so used to wearing it, that when we're older we find we CAN'T leave the house without it!

REASONS FOR WEARING MAKE-UP ...

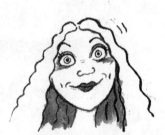

... To look older ...

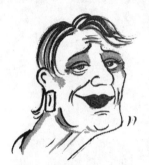

... to look younger ...

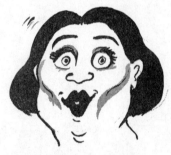

... to look thinner ...

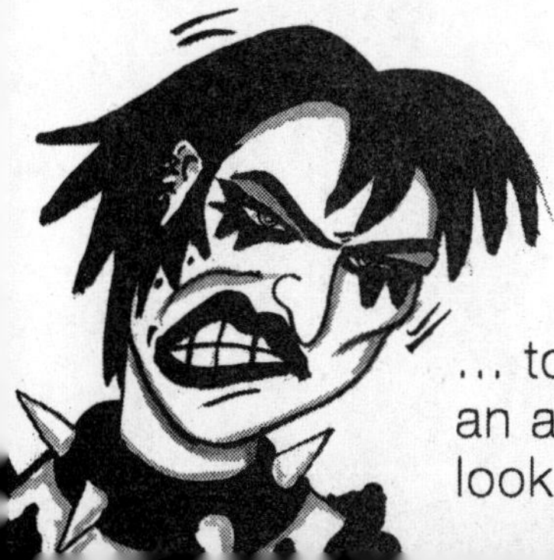

... to give you an aggressive look ...

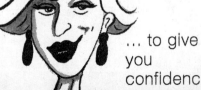

... to give you confidence ...

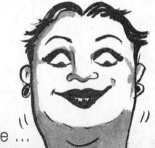

... to give you a CHIN!

Most of the time people are telling us something about themselves by the way they do their make-up.

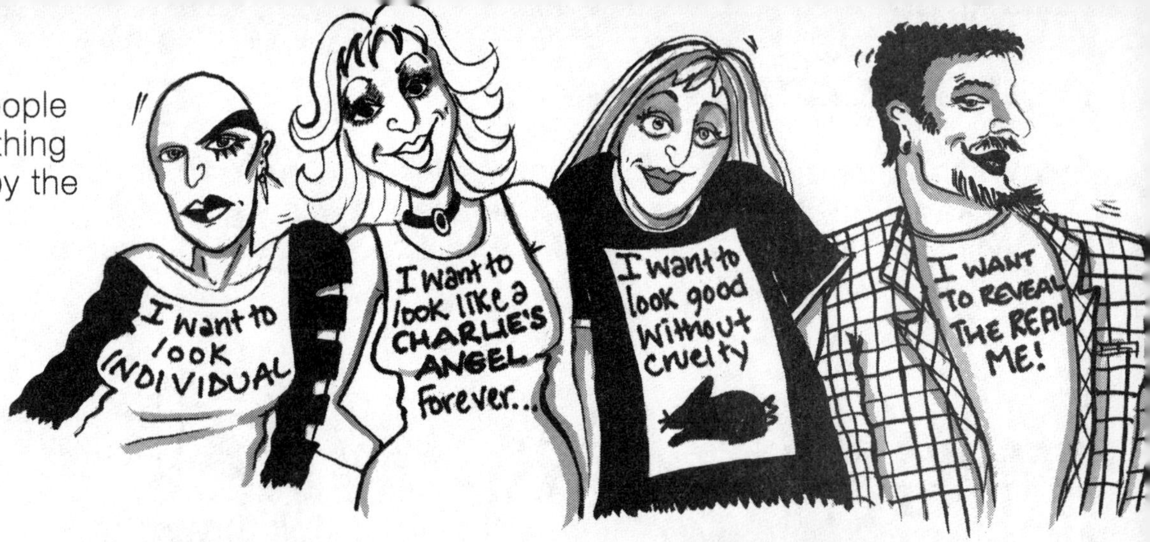
I want to look INDIVIDUAL
I want to look like a CHARLIE'S ANGEL Forever...
I want to look good without cruelty
I WANT TO REVEAL THE REAL ME!

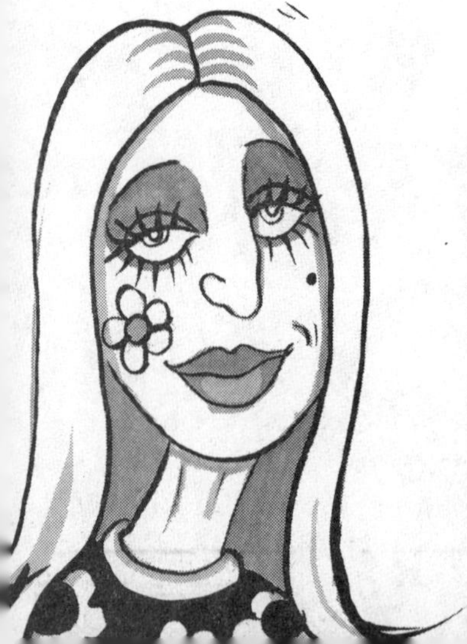

Unfortunately, sometimes the only thing they're telling us is that they haven't changed the way they do their make-up since they were teenagers. (Especially noticeable if you were a swinger in the sixties.)

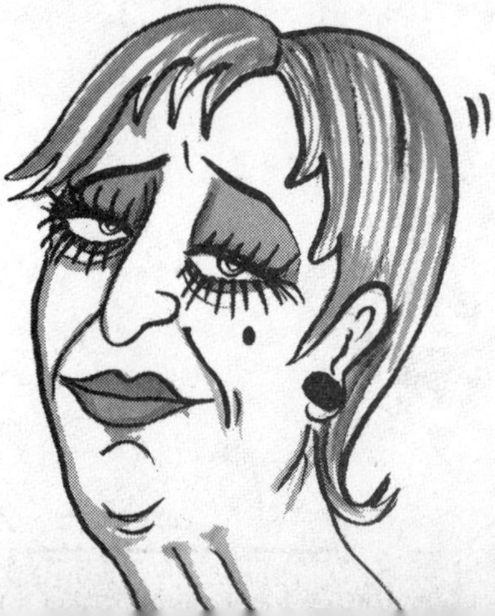

MAKE-UP MISTAKES ...

We've all been there. The day when you know you did your make-up too quickly, or just plain BADLY. When it happens to other people it's very entertaining, but not so hot when it's happening to *you*!

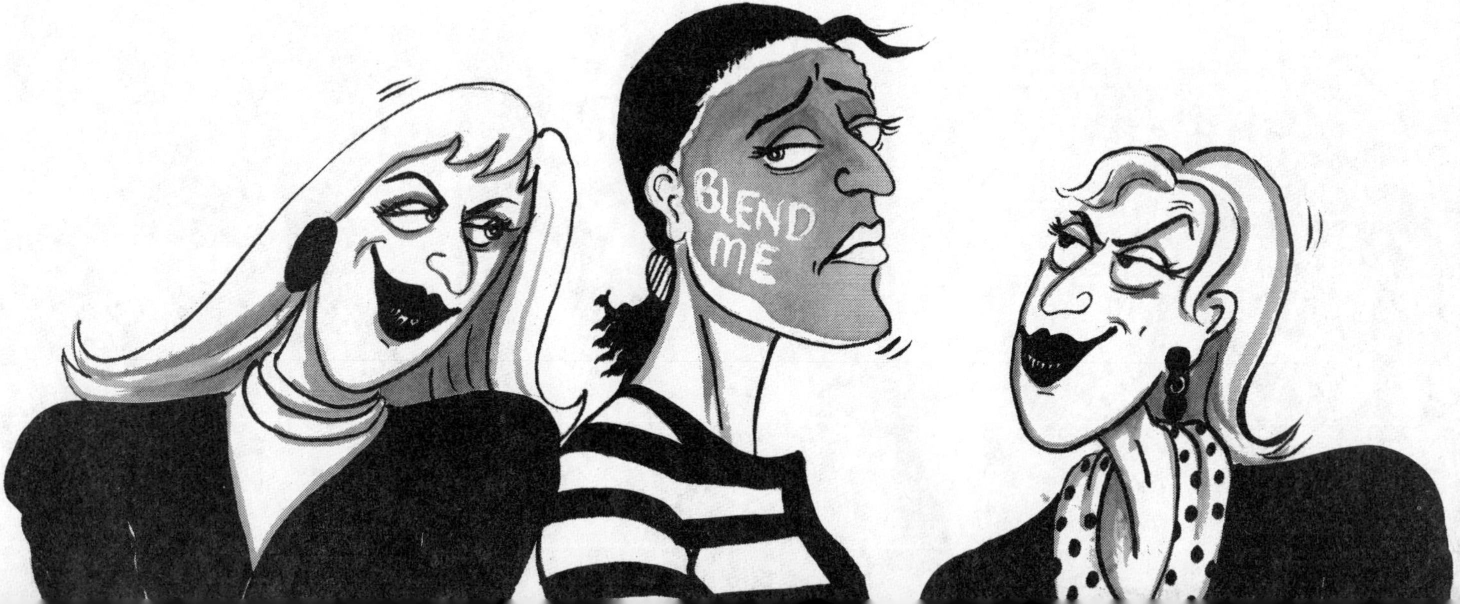
BLEND ME

The most frequent mistakes we make are with foundation ...

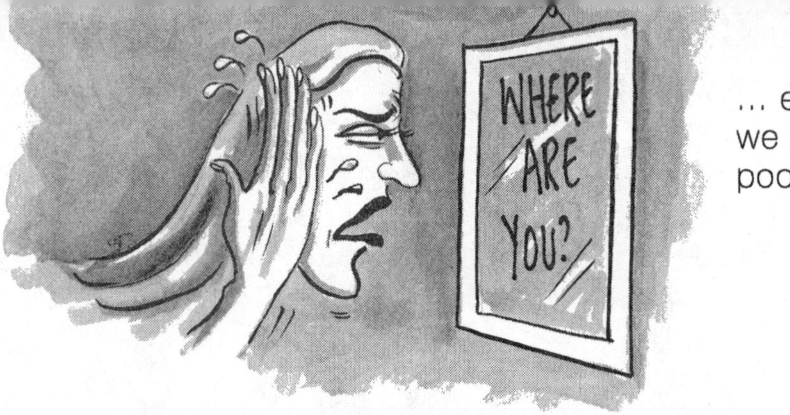
WHERE ARE YOU?

... especially if we put it on in a poor light.

It always ends up looking too heavy ...

... too pale ...

... or completely the WRONG COLOUR!

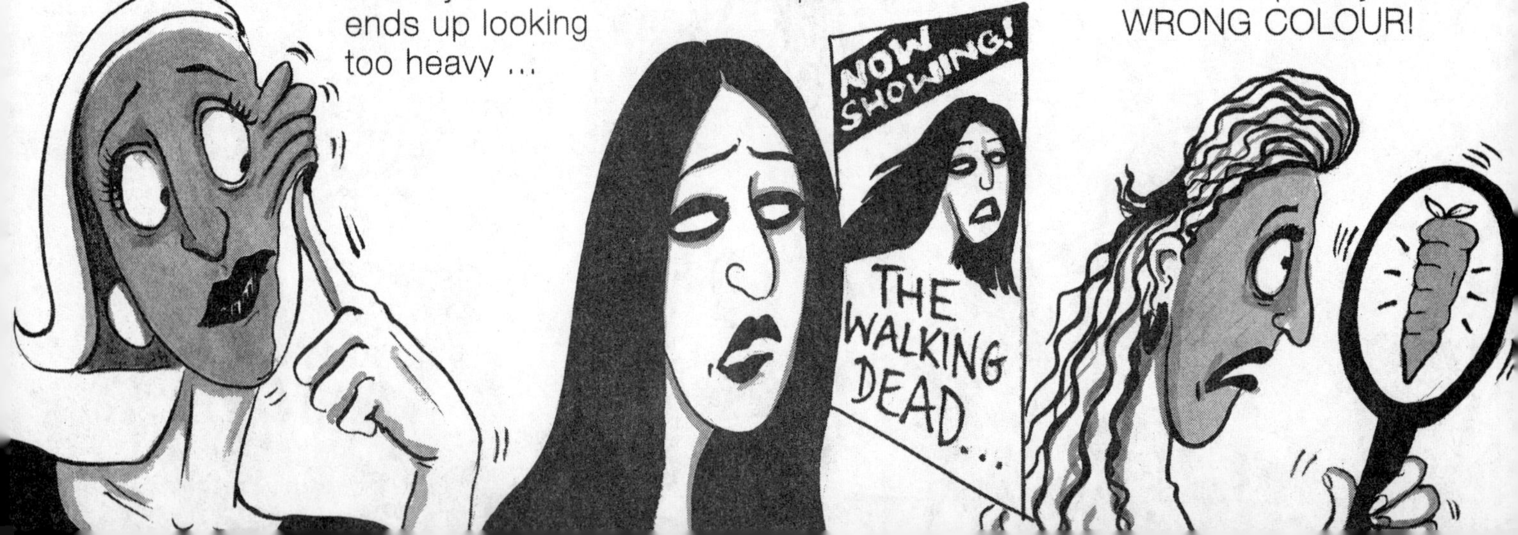
NOW SHOWING!
THE WALKING DEAD...

Tell-Tale signs that it's gone horribly wrong ...

People mistake your blusher for a bruise ...

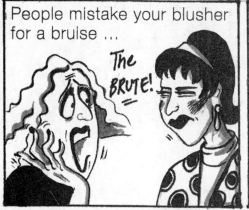

... when people talk to you they look at your smudge ...

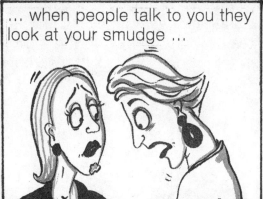

... they rub parts of their face ...

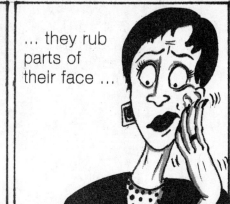

... and start to bring "make-up mistakes I have known" into the conversation.

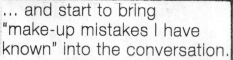
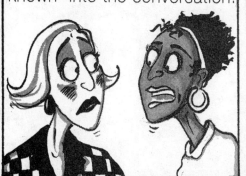

But the most screamingly obvious mistake is when your face is a totally different colour to your neck.

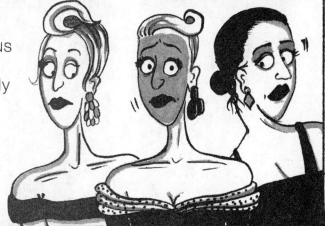

It's not surprising that we make so many mistakes. We buy make-up from shops that have ghastly lighting, there never seems to be a tester when you want one, and as soon as you find a perfect product ... it gets discontinued.

And life gets even more frustrating when your skin shade doesn't match the shade card of the manufacturers.

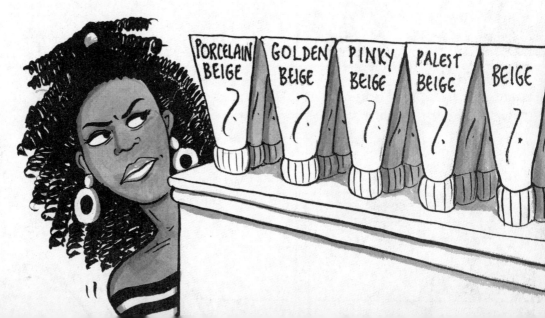

PORCELAIN BEIGE ?

GOLDEN BEIGE ?

PINKY BEIGE ?

PALEST BEIGE ?

BEIGE ?

The one thing about large shops that is (almost) enough to put you off make-up for life are the lipstick-smirking, foundation-slapping, mascara-laden sample-spraying SALES GIRLS!

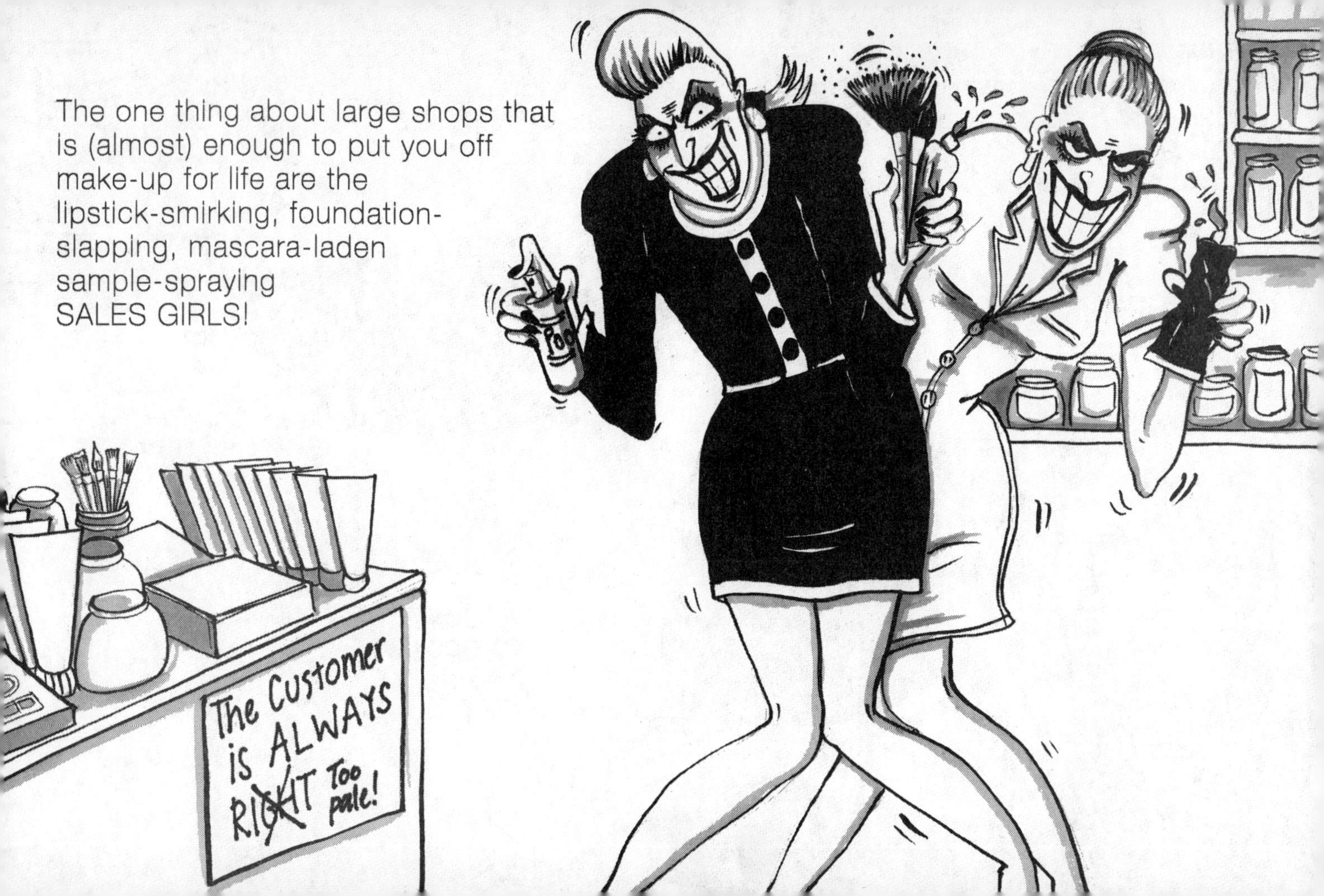

Too
The Customer is ALWAYS RIGHT
Too pale!

If they don't have your eye out with their latest perfume samples, they do their best to lure you onto their counter ...

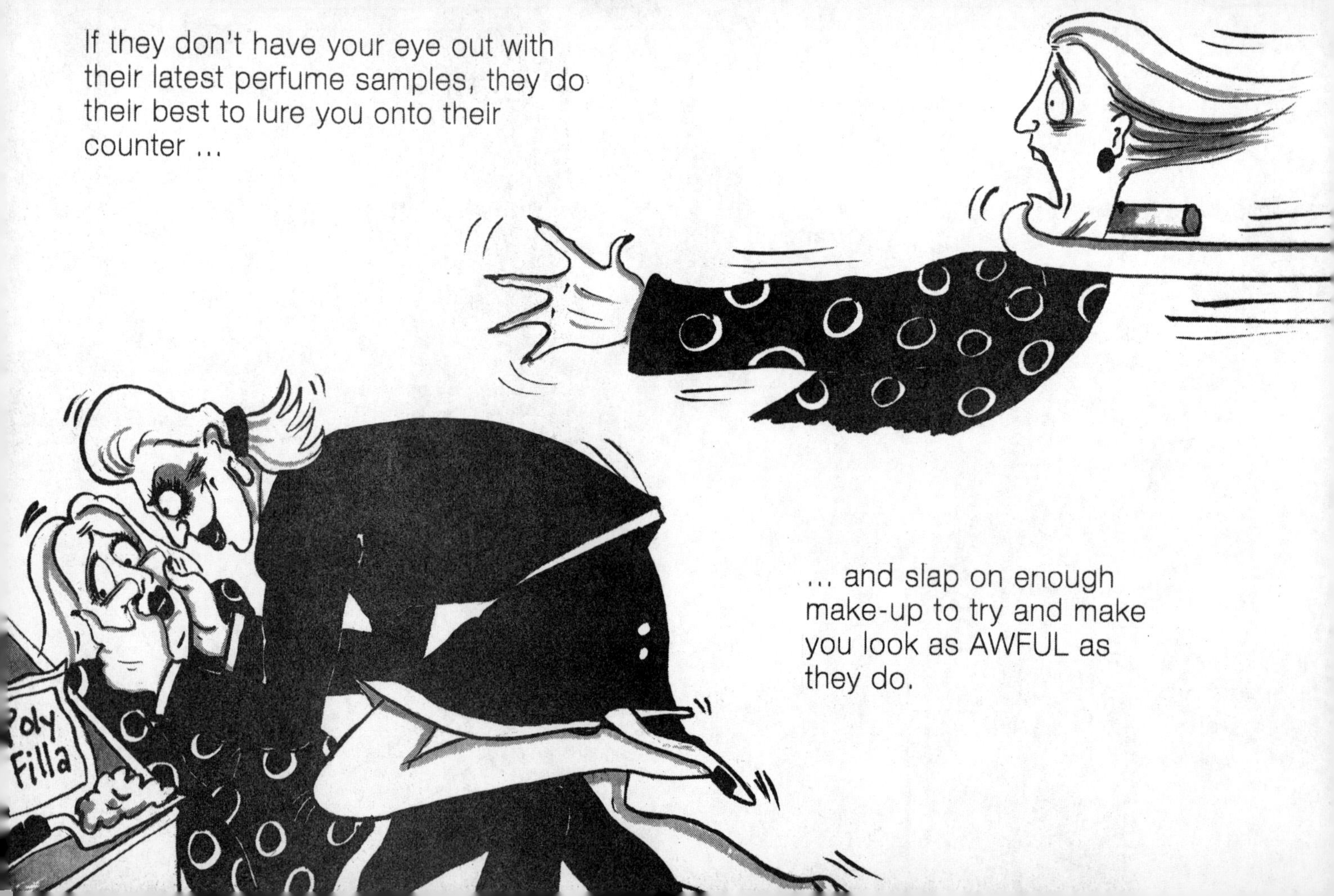
Poly
Filla

... and slap on enough make-up to try and make you look as AWFUL as they do.

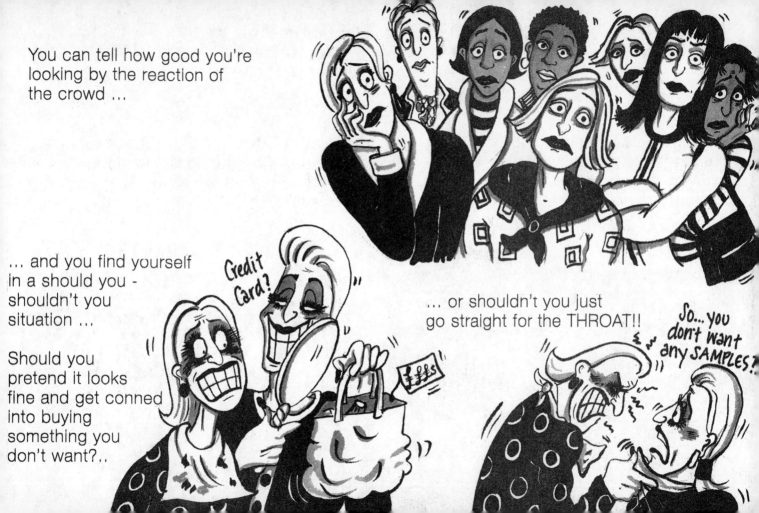

You can tell how good you're looking by the reaction of the crowd ...

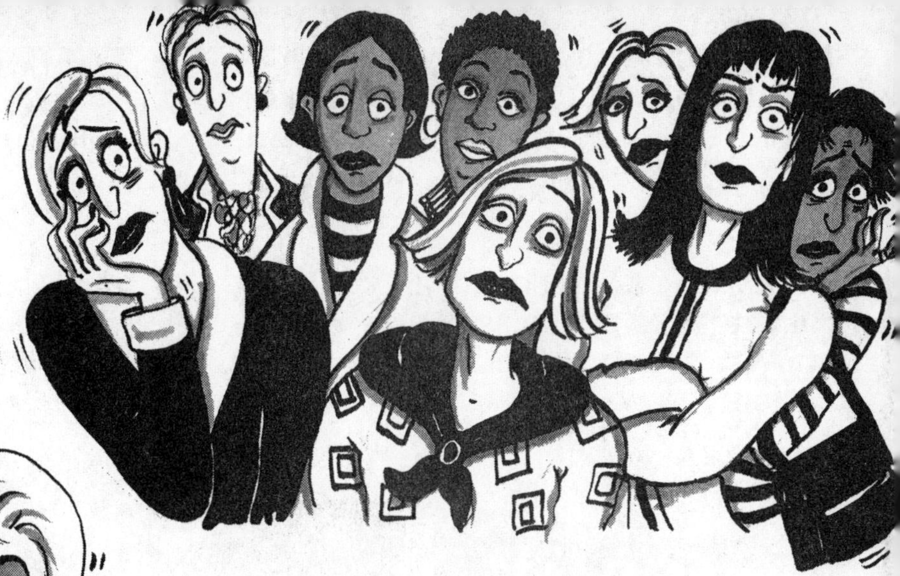

... and you find yourself in a should you - shouldn't you situation ...

Should you pretend it looks fine and get conned into buying something you don't want?..

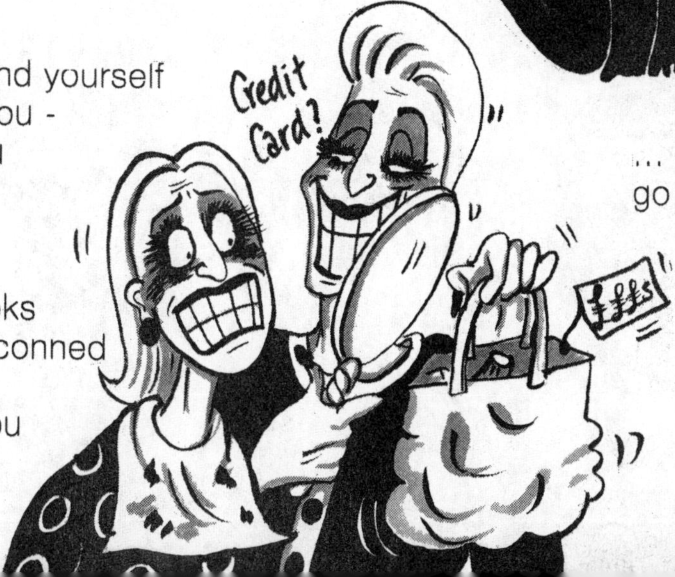
Credit Card?
£££s

... or shouldn't you just go straight for the THROAT!!

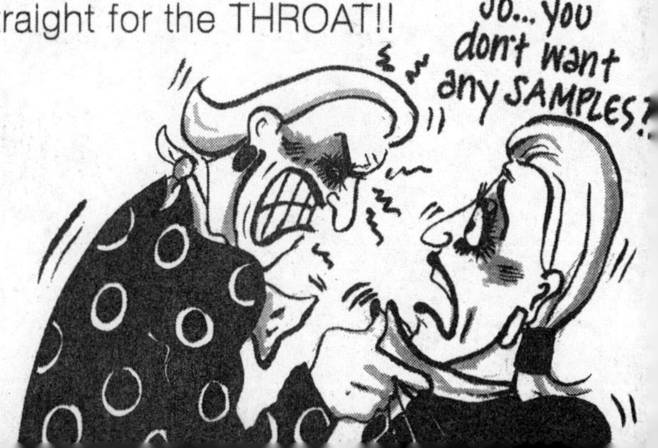
So... you don't want any SAMPLES?!

TANNING: Since frazzling your skin to bits for two weeks a year was finally declared BAD for you, we have been searching for an effective alternative that won't turn us orange or kill us.

SUN BEDS are expensive, aren't guaranteed to protect your skin, and they make you feel like a toasted sandwich.

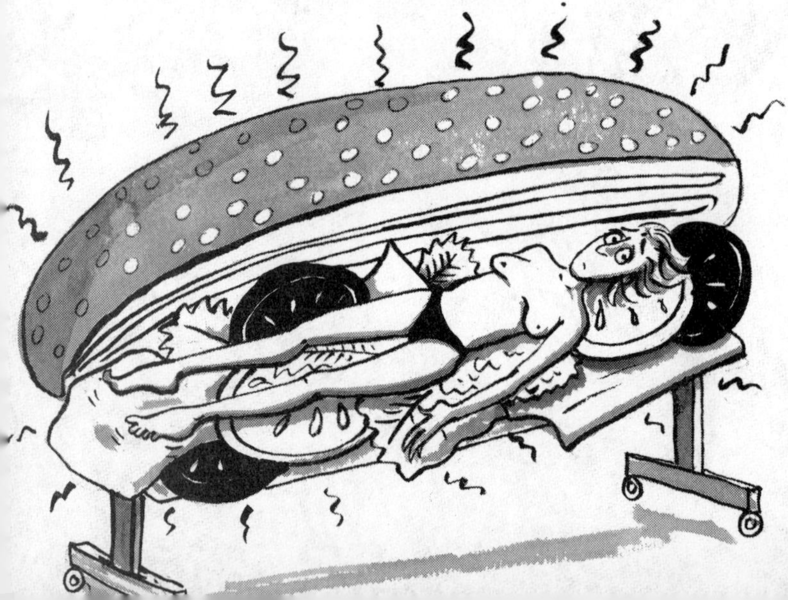

Taking a TANNING PILL sounds far too risky. Call me old fashioned, but I believe you should get your suntan from the OUTSIDE.

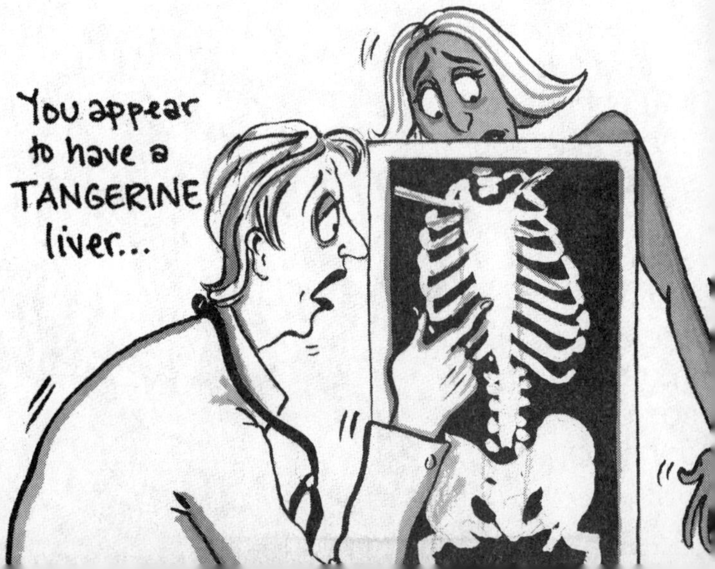
You appear to have a TANGERINE liver...

Cheap and cheerful products include
LEG MAKE-UP, which is a cosmetic
equivalent to the tea-bag staining
the old girls used to do in the war.
It's fine, as long as you don't go
out in the rain or cross your legs ... *ever!*

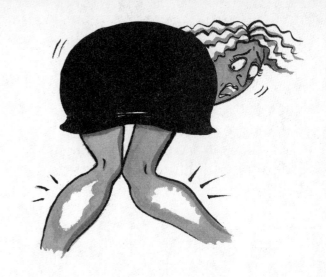

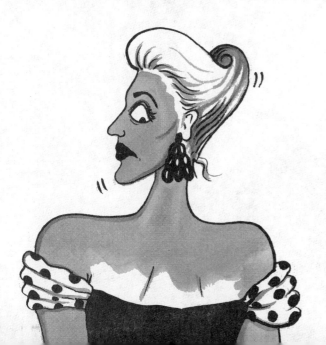

The best types of fake tan are those
that come out after 3 hours, and
last for days. As it doesn't wash
out quickly it's a good idea to rub
it in properly.

HAIR REMOVAL ...

Now, Continental women and Hippies can say what they like, but displaying bushes of hair in your armpits and growing forests on your legs is about as attractive as ... well, a MOUSTACHE!

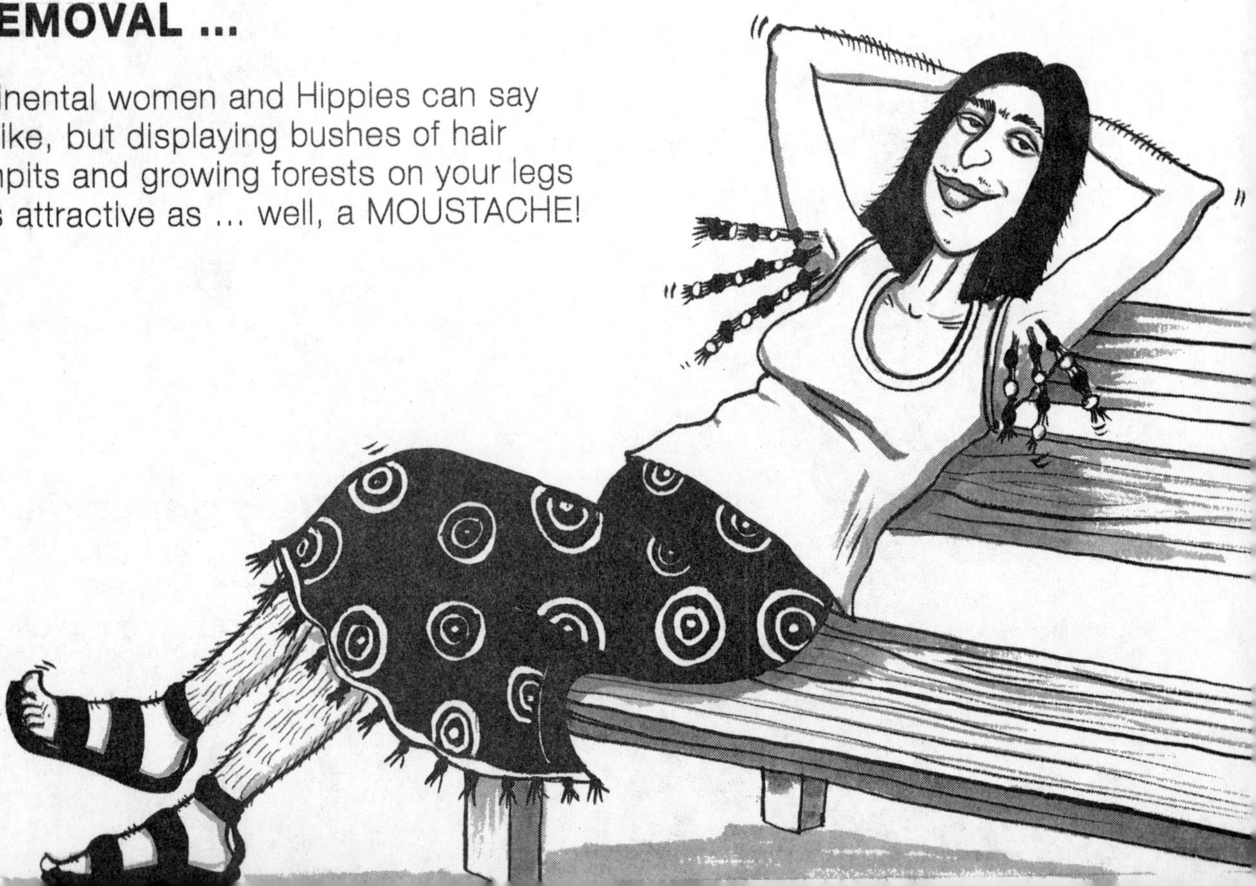

Our mothers warn us that once
we start shaving, our hairs
grow back twice as thick, and
we have to keep doing it
forever. Scarey stuff alright,
... but WHO CARES?

I think we all have a go at
plucking our hairs out with
tweezers. We never stick to it,
mainly because it's boring,
but also because we can't
bear to do it to our *armpits!*

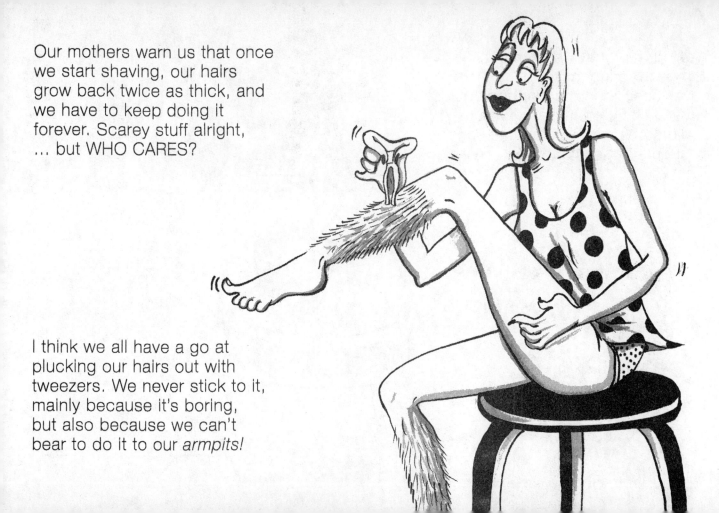

Waxing at home is something I can never bring myself to do. I've never been fond of pain, and could never inflict it on myself. (I also couldn't manage to grow the hairs to such a huge length.)

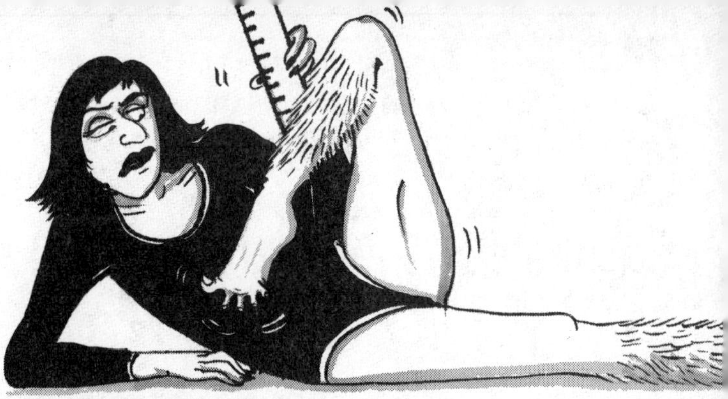

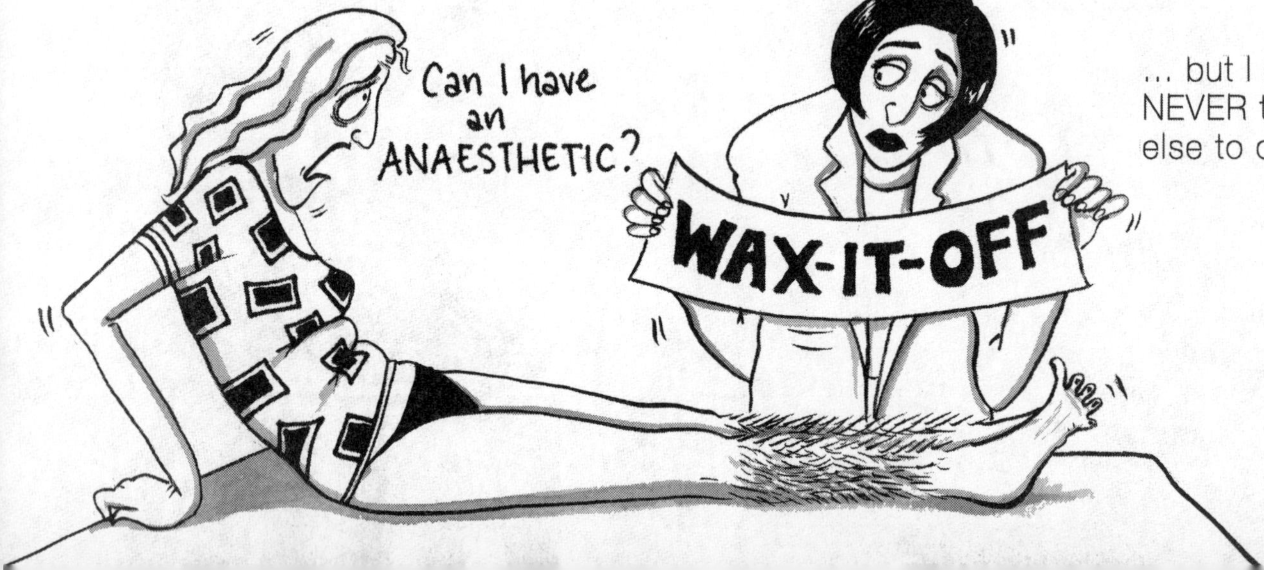
Can I have an ANAESTHETIC?
WAX-IT-OFF

... but I could NEVER trust anyone else to do it.

Hair removing cream is smelly, awkward and messy ... and you can *guarantee* the doorbell will ring as soon as you put it on ...

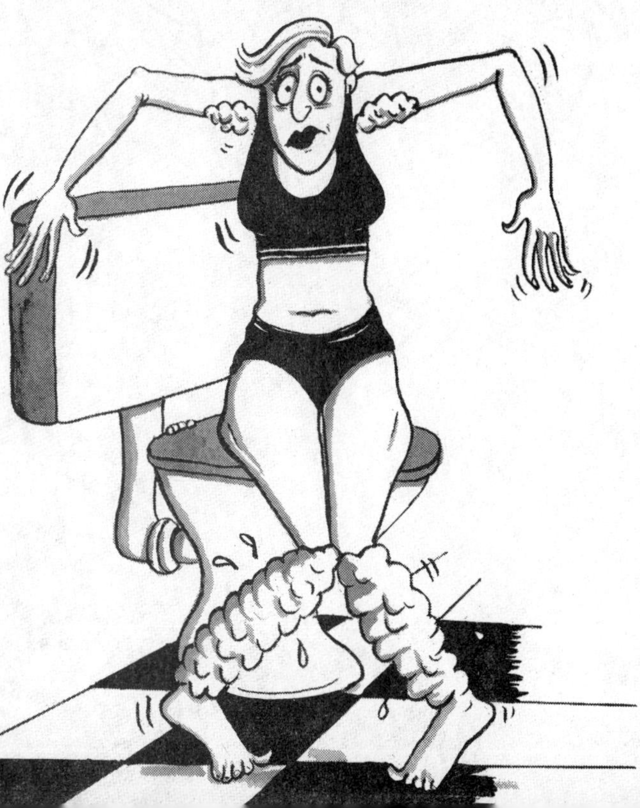

... and Electrolysis just sounds far too SURGICAL!

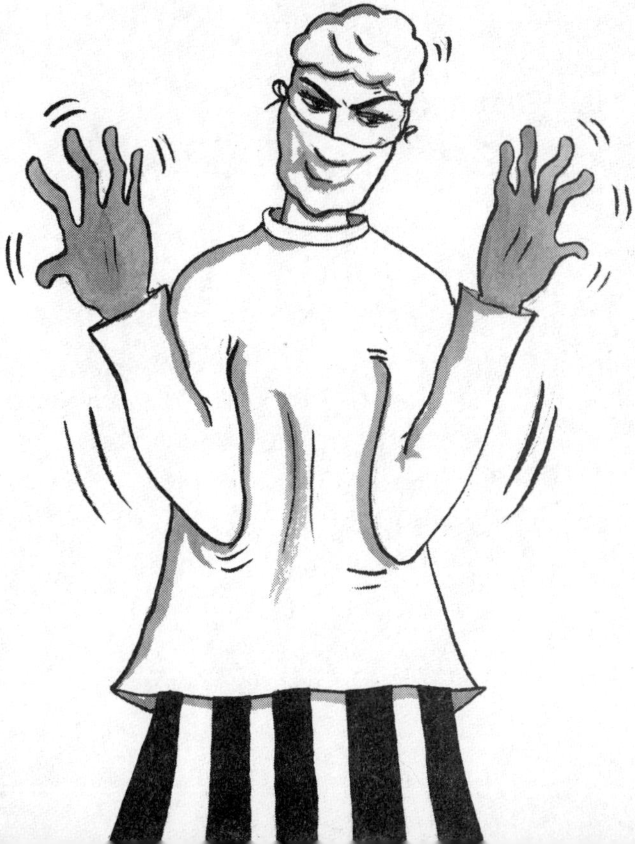

Strangely, men aren't
supposed to like seeing
us in the act of
Hair Removal.

— Does it shatter our Feminine Mystique?
— Do they think we get these
   oh-so-silky legs by magic?
— Or is it because they just can't
   bear to see us using their RAZORS??

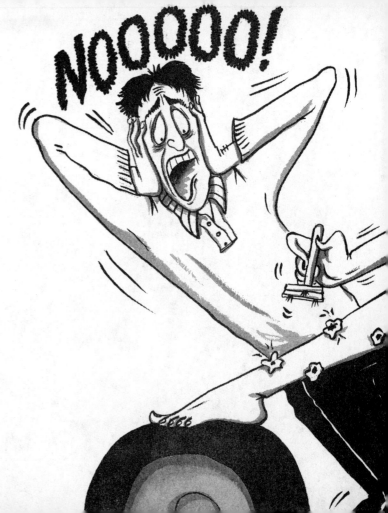

HAIR

TRUST ME

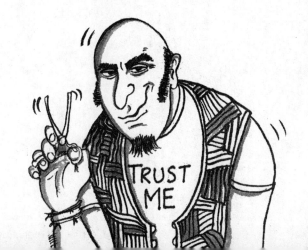

HAIRCUT FROM HELL!

Our hair is our most precious asset; mainly because if our hair goes wrong it's the quickest way for us to look like DOGS.

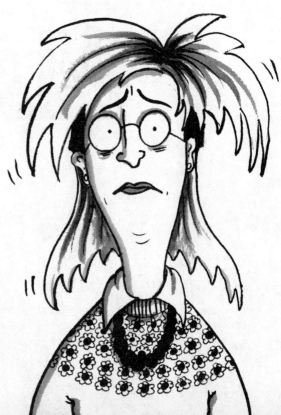

Why then, do we trust our friends to perm our hair?..

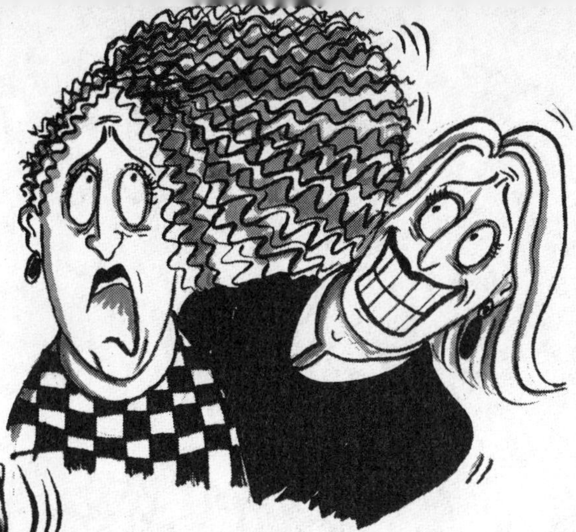
It's quite nice, really...

Why do we take stupid risks to try and LIGHTEN it?..

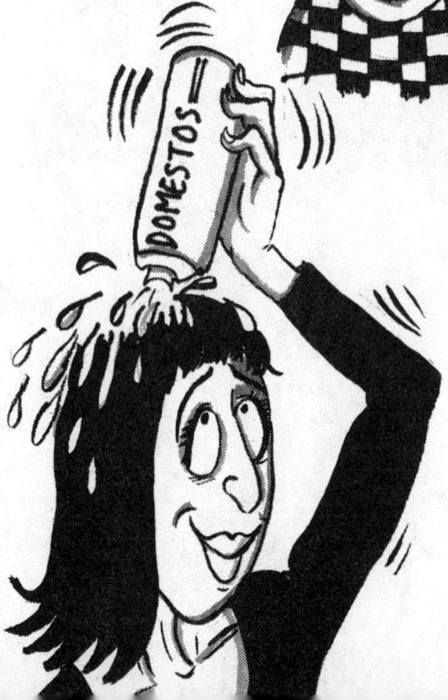
DOMESTOS

... and why ... WHY do we keep cutting it OURSELVES?

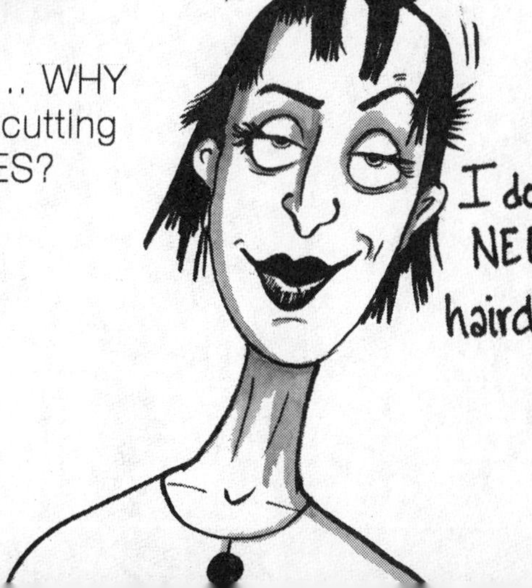
I don't NEED hairdressers.

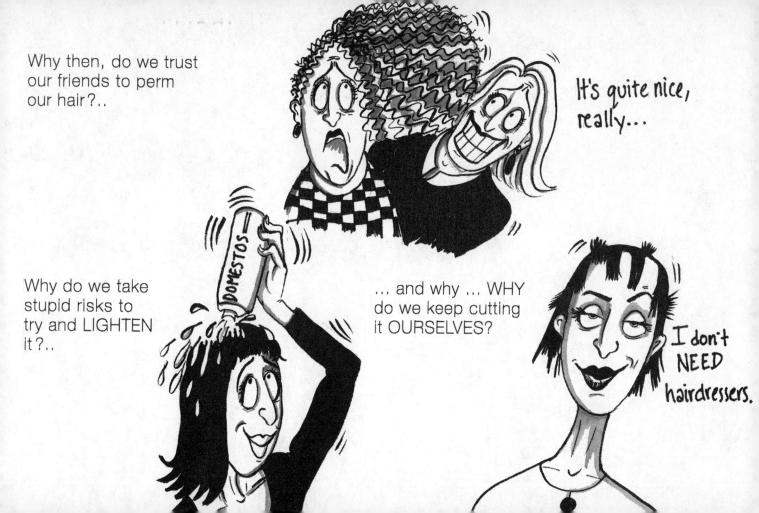

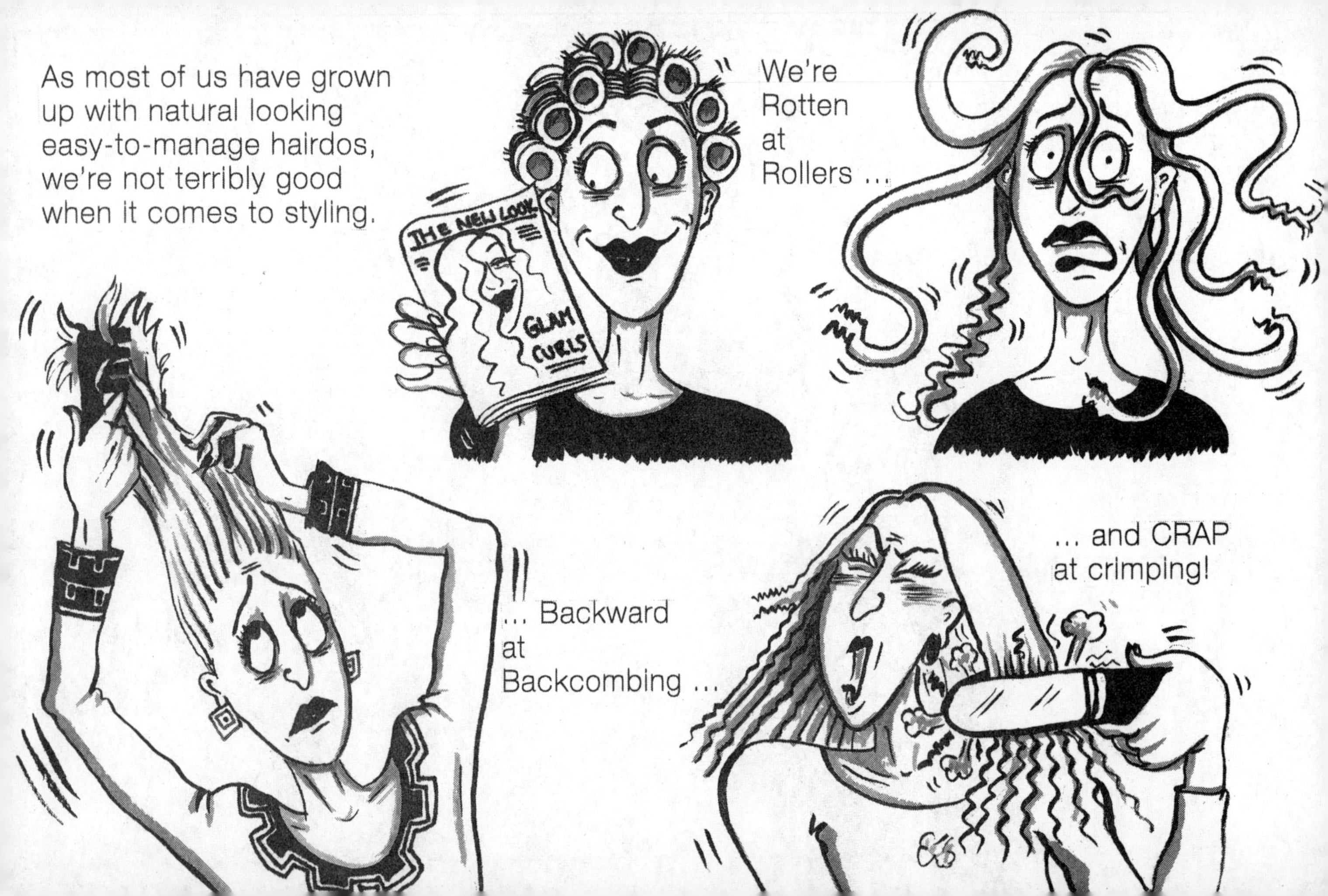
As most of us have grown up with natural looking easy-to-manage hairdos, we're not terribly good when it comes to styling.
THE NEW LOOK
GLAM CURLS
We're Rotten at Rollers ...
... Backward at Backcombing ...
... and CRAP at crimping!

... And we're not exactly MARVELLOUS with MOUSSE!

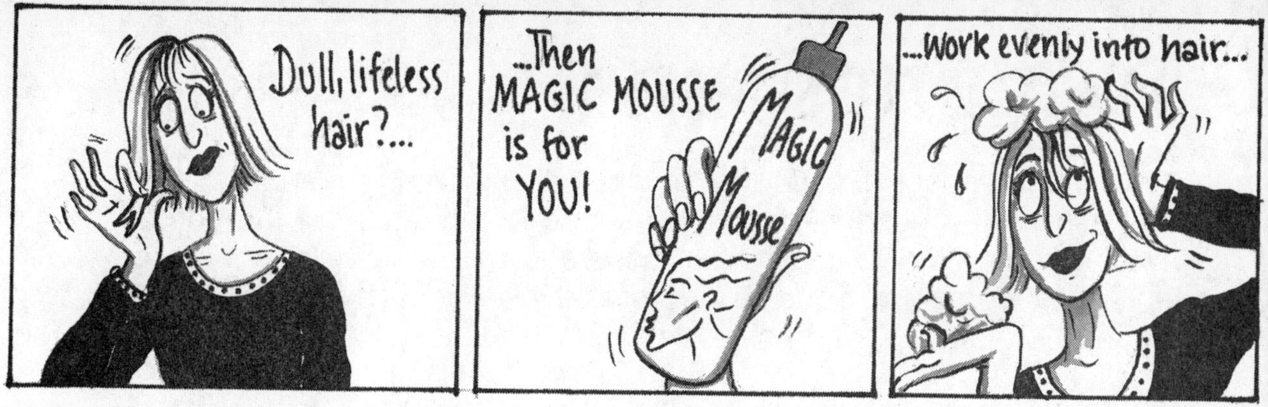
Dull, lifeless hair?...
...Then MAGIC MOUSSE is for YOU!
MAGIC Mousse
...Work evenly into hair...

No wonder we give in and go to HAIRDRESSERS!

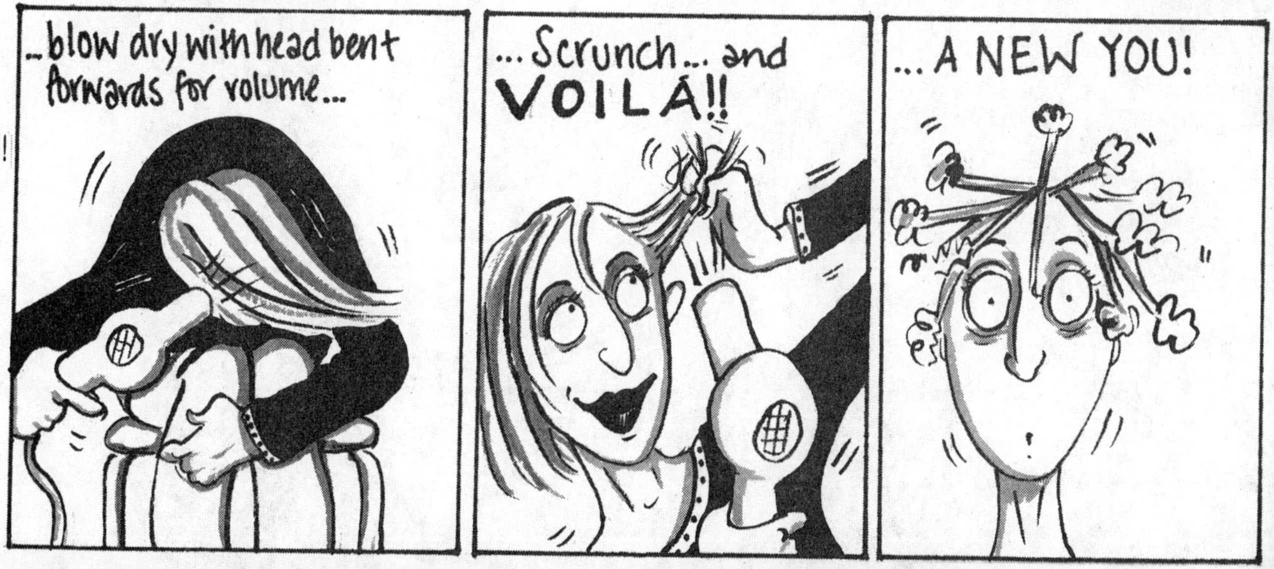
..blow dry with head bent forwards for volume...
... Scrunch... and VOILÁ!!
... A NEW YOU!

HAIRDRESSERS:

As the hairdresser pins you to the chair and looms in brandishing his scissors, the experience is very close to the agony of the doctor's waiting room. We go to the hairdressers to get a marvellous-looking style that we couldn't possibly do ourselves ... but if you walk into the salon and the stylists look like something from the Rocky Horror Show ... can you TRUST THEM?

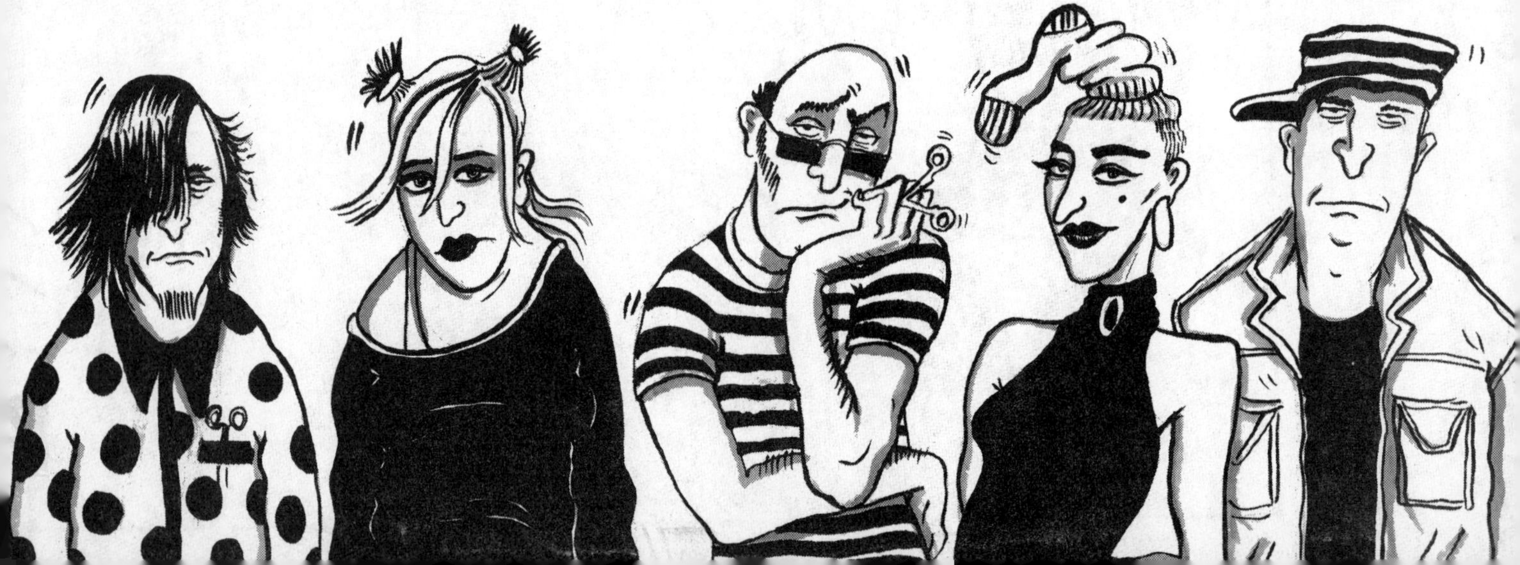

A simple slip to a hairdresser can be a complete disaster to you. All you can think about is how long it's going to take to grow it out. All they can think about is how quickly they can get you out of the salon.

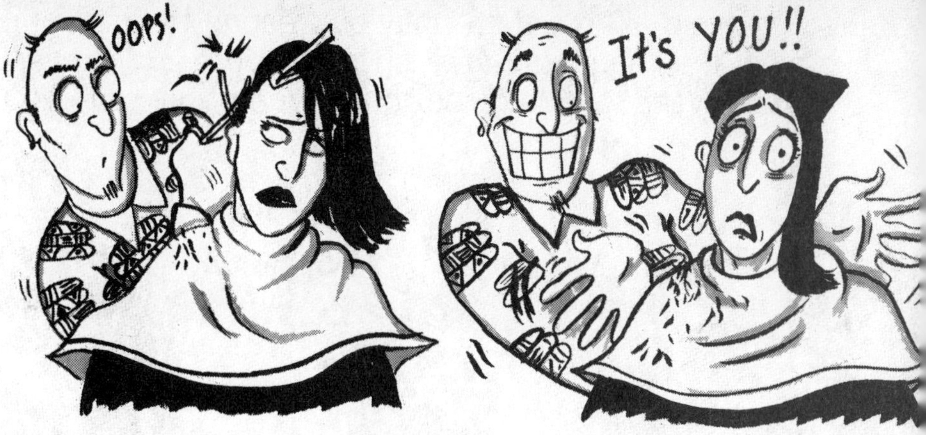
OOPS!
It's YOU!!

The real problem arises because they treat their hair as an accessory and are constantly changing their image. No wonder a few inches here and there don't seem too traumatic.

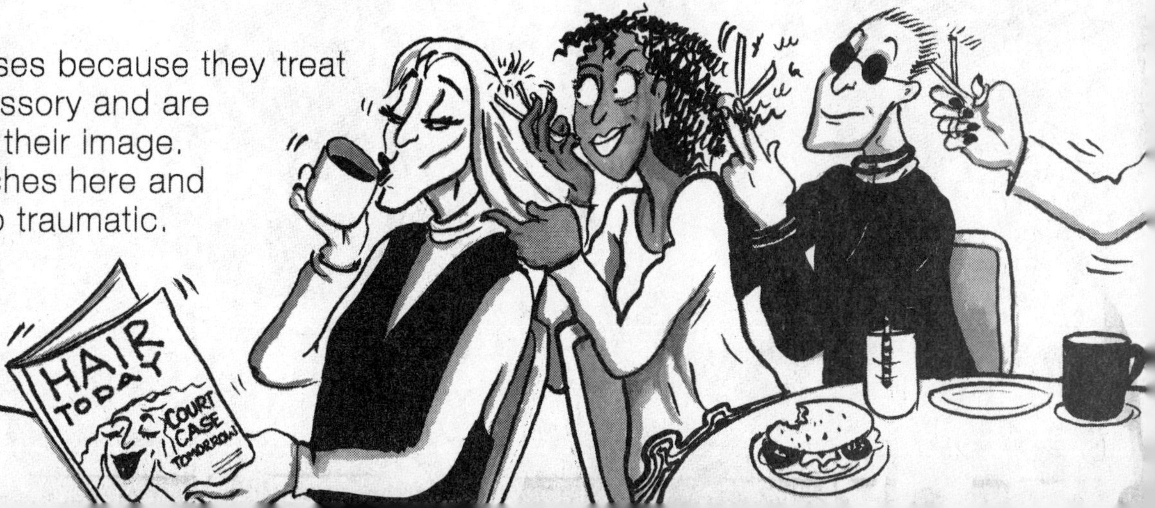
HAIR TODAY
COURT CASE TOMORROW

Try to avoid all risk of calamity by wearing the sort of clothes that project the image you think suits you best. Hairdressers often take what you are wearing as a guide to the type of hairstyle you need.

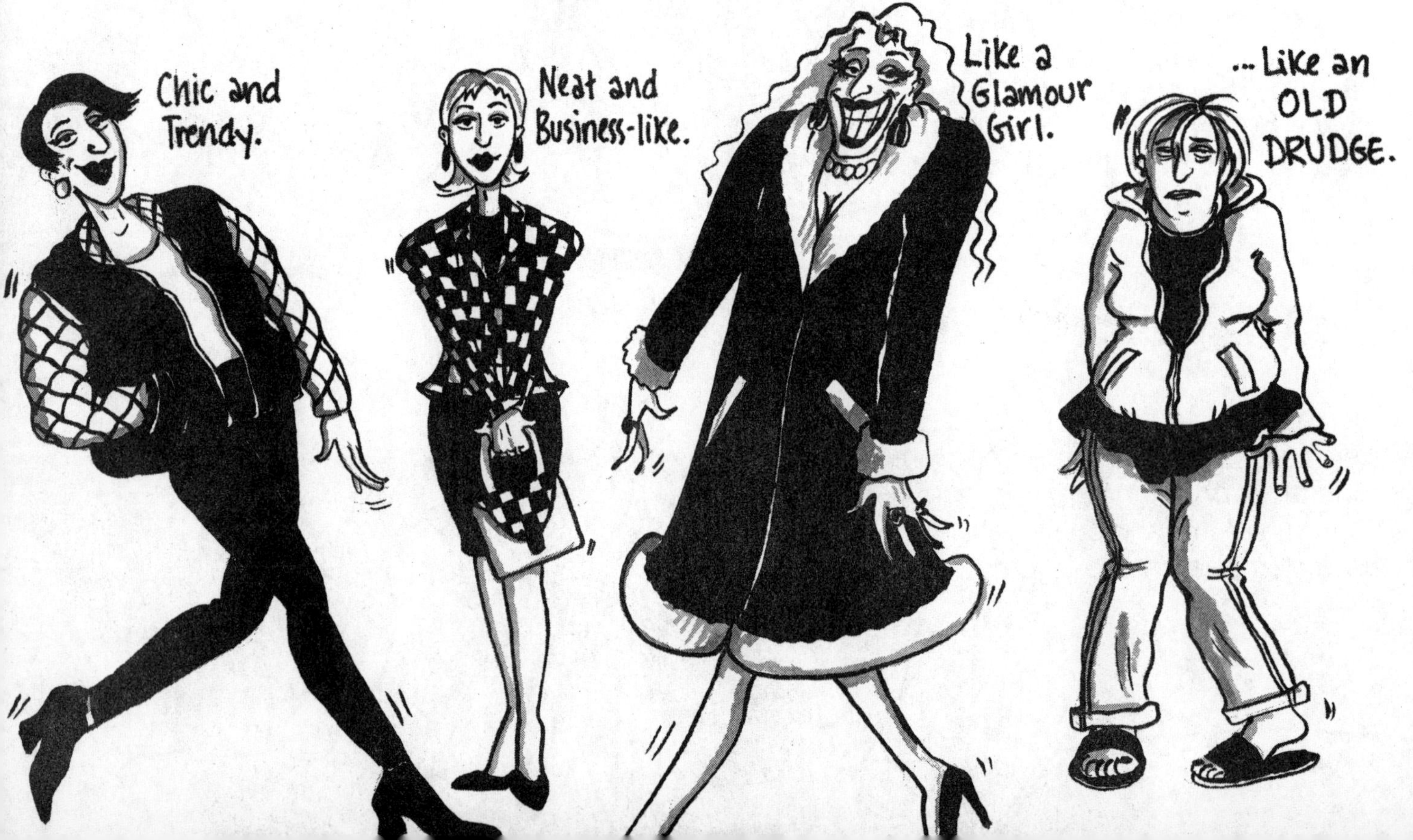

Chic and Trendy.
Neat and Business-like.
Like a Glamour Girl.
...Like an OLD DRUDGE.

When you arrive at the salon, watch out for how other clients look when they come out. It'll give you an idea of how you might end up.

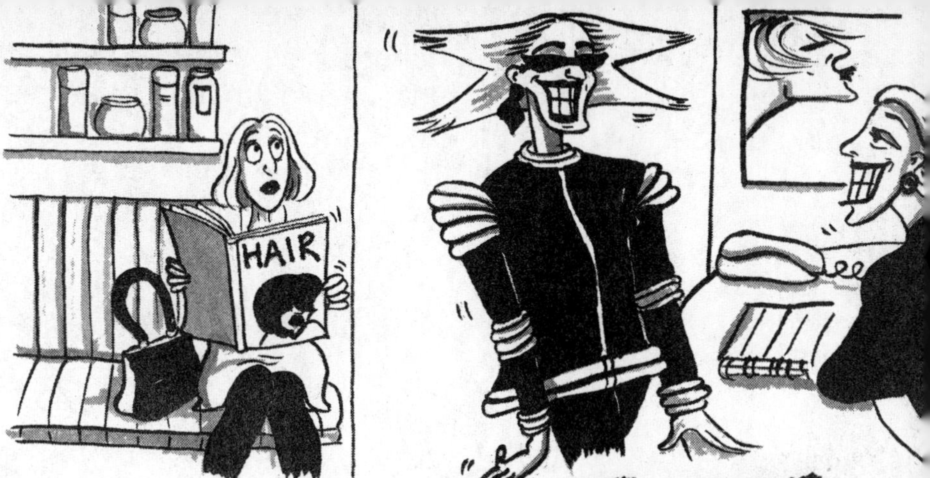
HAIR

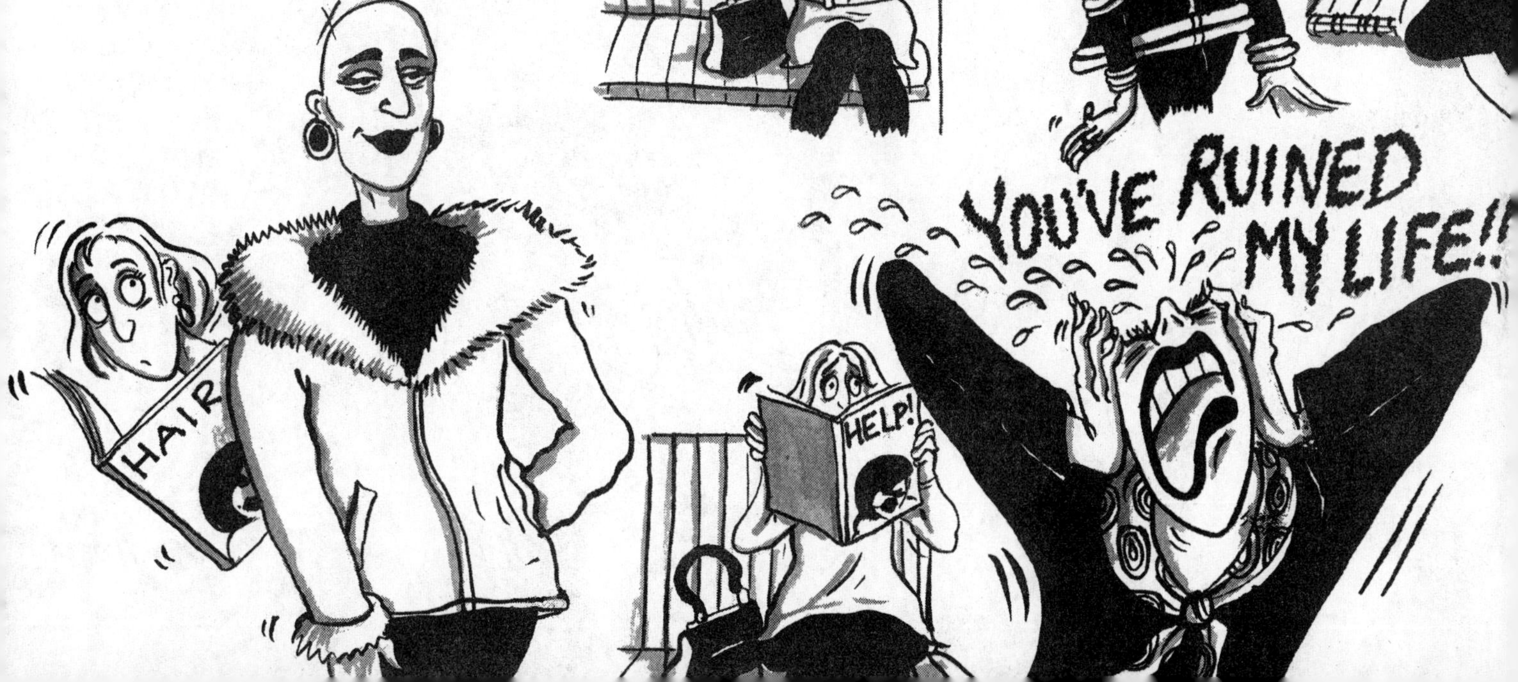
HAIR
HELP!
YOU'VE RUINED MY LIFE!!

The main problem between hairdressers and clients is a total communication breakdown. We say things that we think make perfect sense and are jolly good suggestions, and they look at us as if we were BUFFOONS. As soon as they open their mouths, they begin to speak in an alien tongue. This is because they have been trained in Hairdresser Terminology and have forgotten the days when they knew as little as we do.

WHAT THEY SAY ...

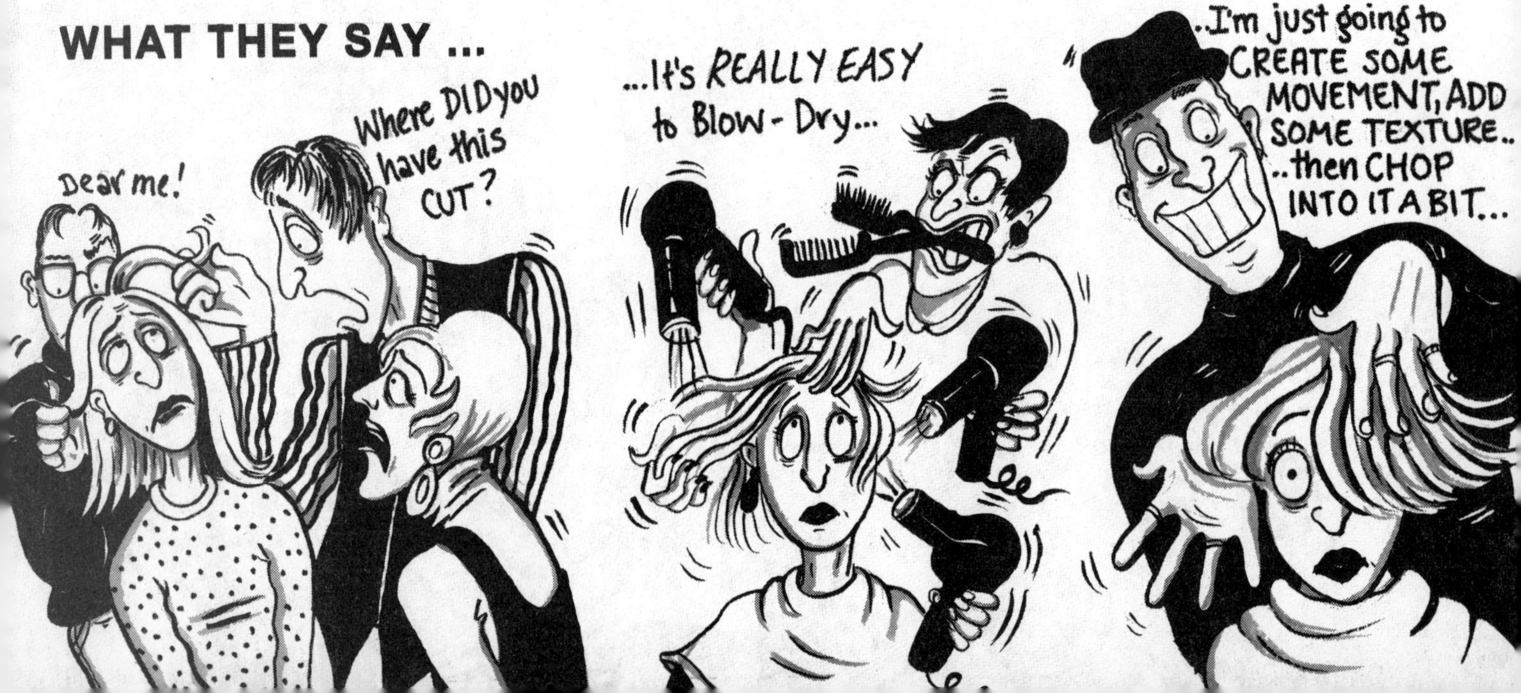
Dear me!
Where DID you have this CUT?
...It's REALLY EASY to Blow-Dry...
"...I'm just going to CREATE SOME MOVEMENT, ADD SOME TEXTURE.. ..then CHOP INTO IT A BIT...

... WHAT WE SAY ...

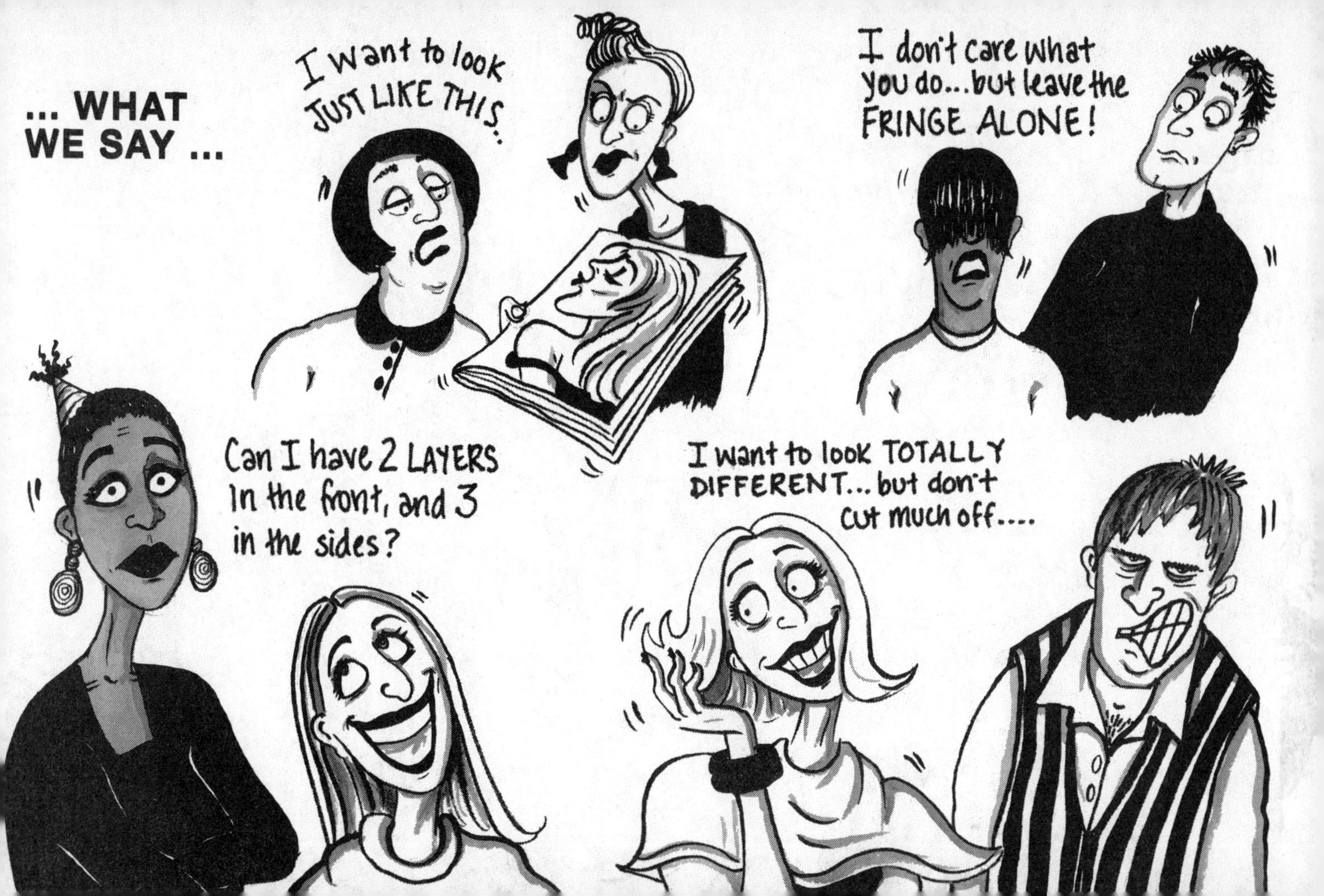
I want to look JUST LIKE THIS...
I don't care what you do...but leave the FRINGE ALONE!
Can I have 2 LAYERS in the front, and 3 in the sides?
I want to look TOTALLY DIFFERENT... but don't cut much off....

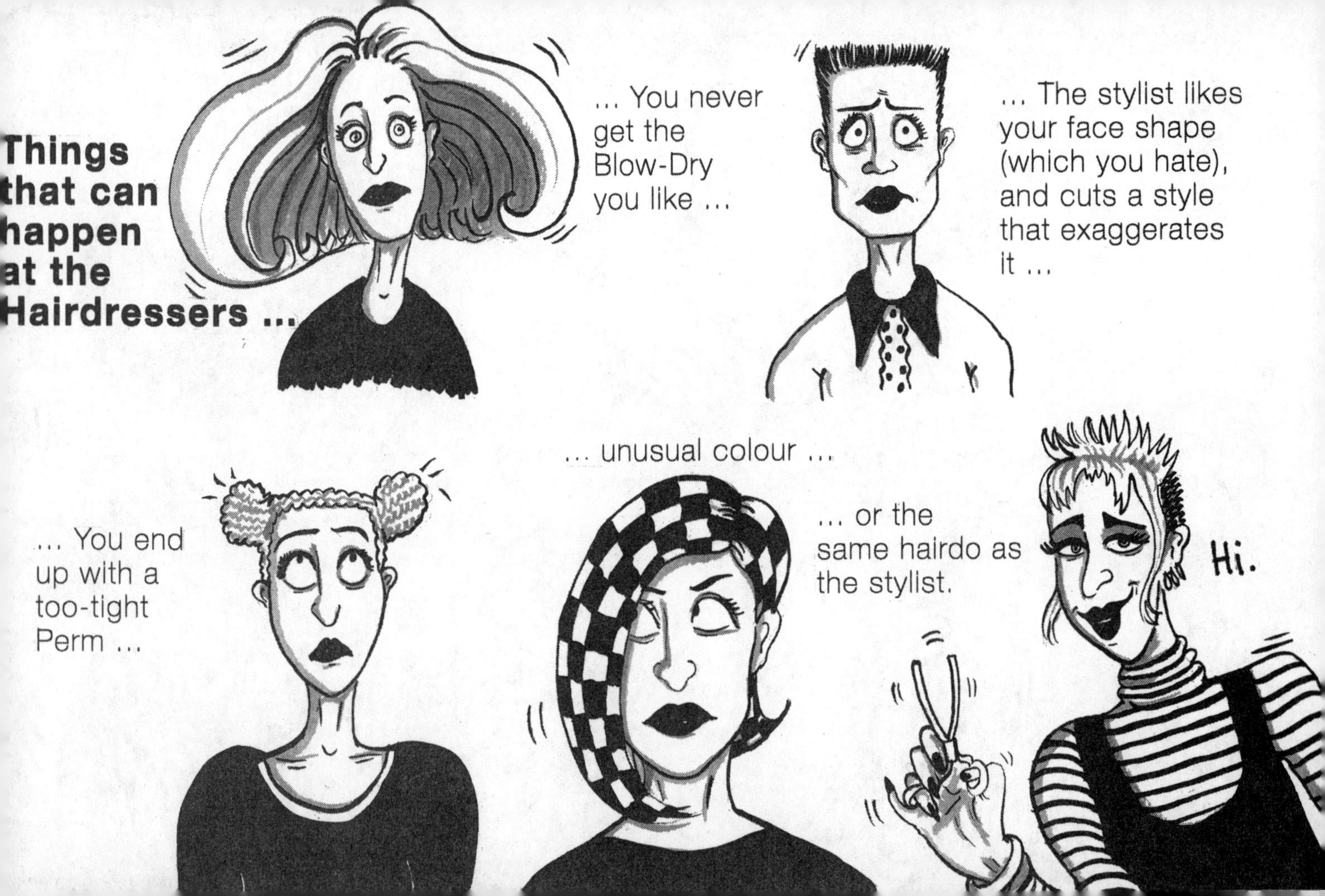
Things that can happen at the Hairdressers ...
... You never get the Blow-Dry you like ...
... The stylist likes your face shape (which you hate), and cuts a style that exaggerates it ...
... You end up with a too-tight Perm ...
... unusual colour ...
... or the same hairdo as the stylist.
Hi.

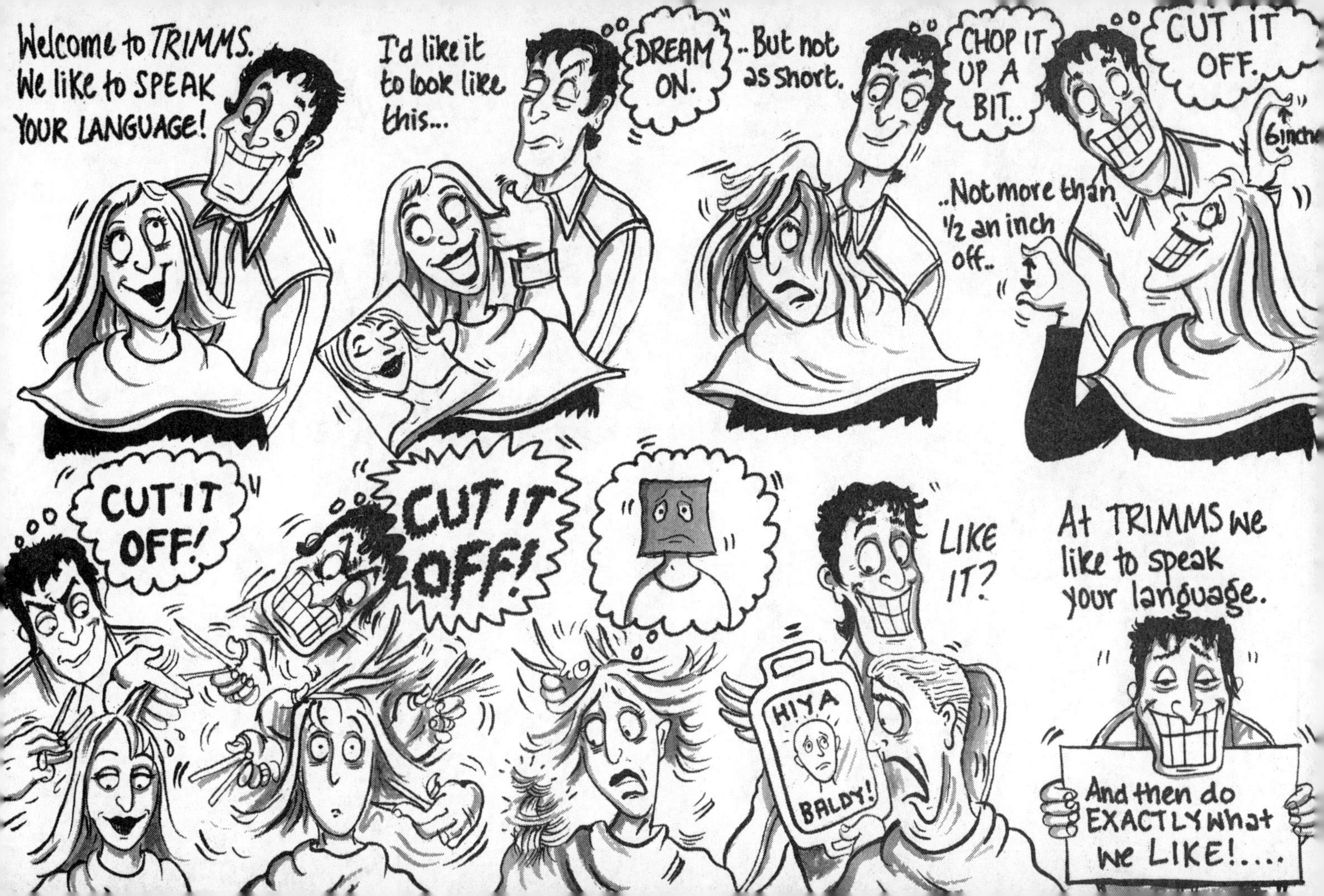
Welcome to TRIMMS. We like to SPEAK YOUR LANGUAGE!
I'd like it to look like this...
DREAM ON.
..But not as short.
CHOP IT UP A BIT..
..Not more than 1/2 an inch off..
CUT IT OFF.
6inche
CUT IT OFF!
CUT IT OFF!
LIKE IT?
HIYA BALDY!
At TRIMMS we like to speak your language.
And then do EXACTLY what we LIKE!....

HOW TO SURVIVE YOUR HAIRDRESSER ...

Wear clothes that reflect the REAL YOU ...

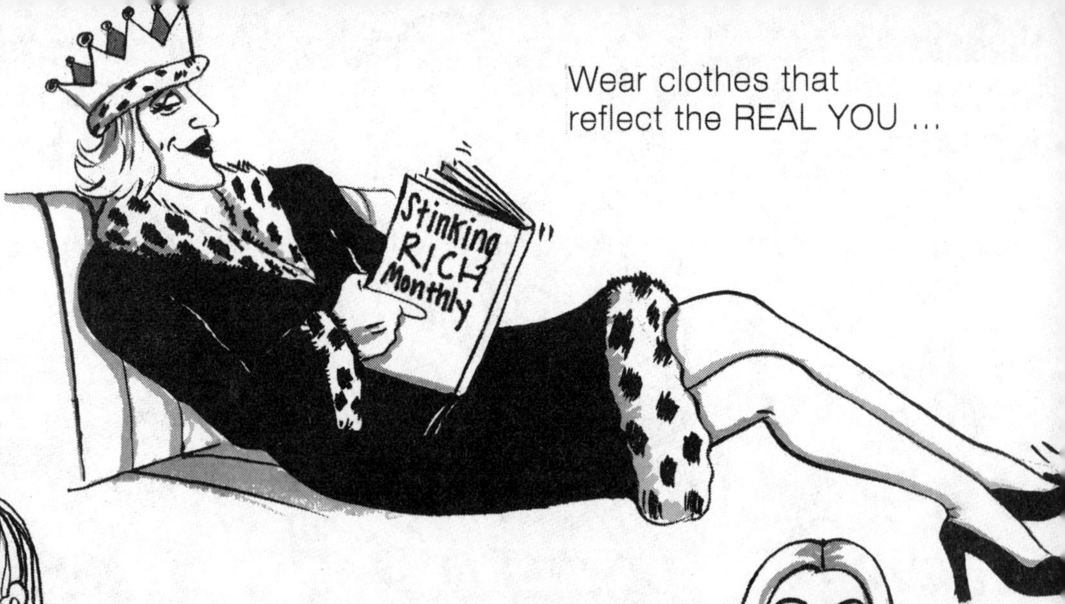
Stinking RICH Monthly

Talk to the stylist at length about what you want ...

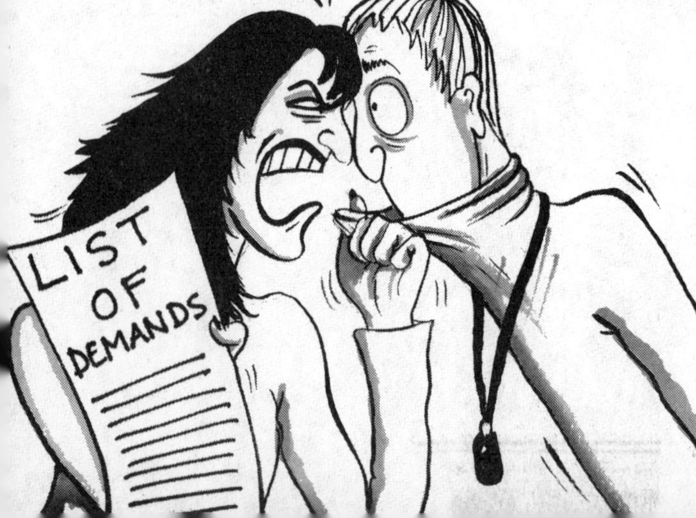
LIST OF DEMANDS

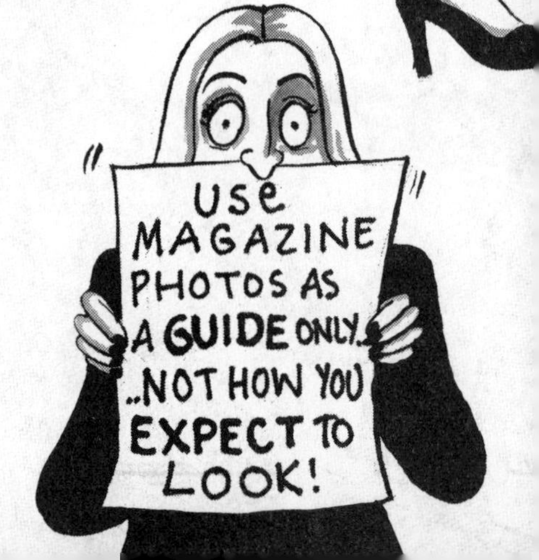
USE MAGAZINE PHOTOS AS A GUIDE ONLY. ..NOT HOW YOU EXPECT TO LOOK!

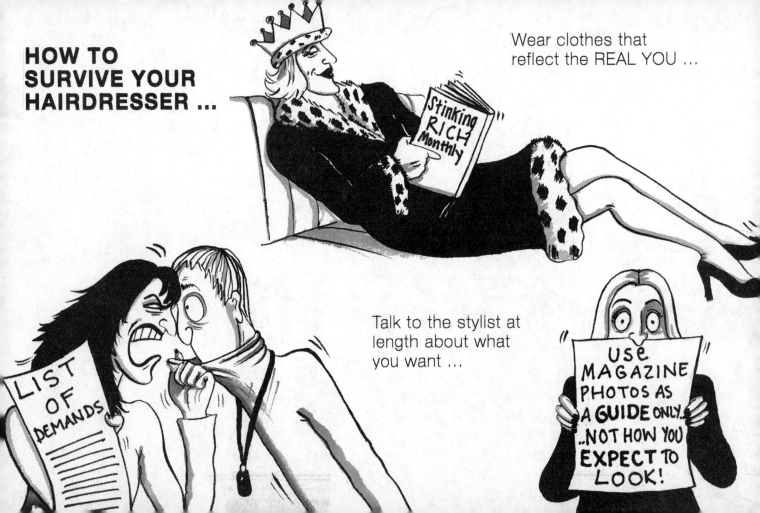

... Keep your eye on how short your hair is getting ...

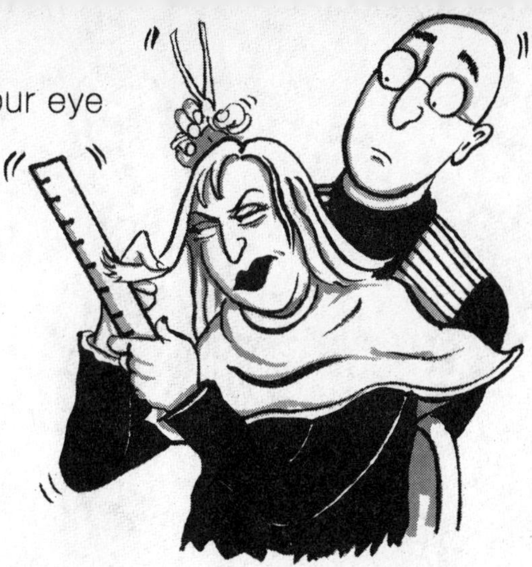

... Ask to be shown how to blow dry it so you can do it at home ...

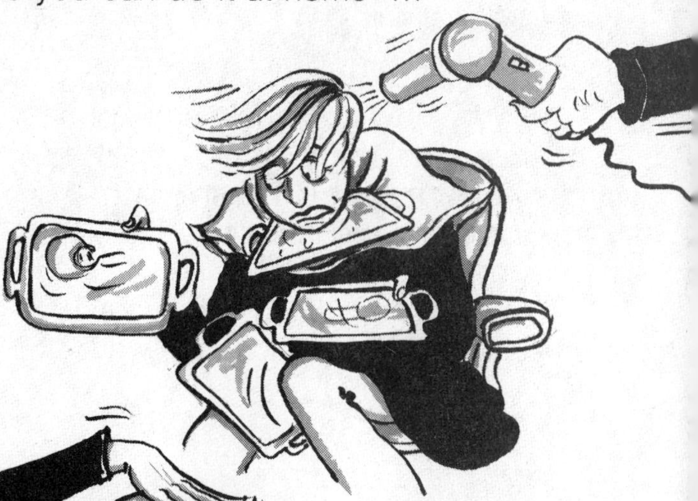

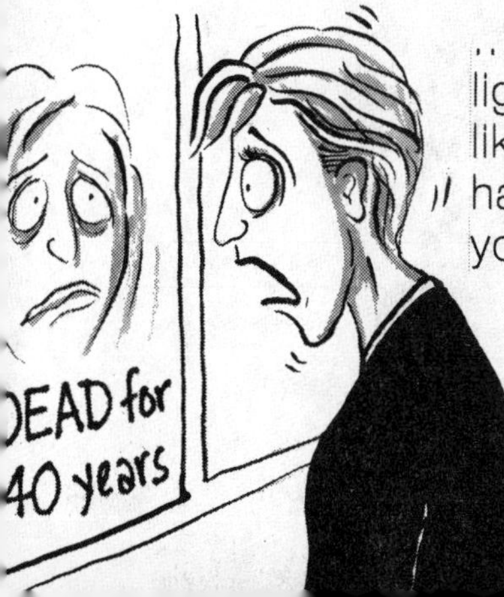
DEAD for
40 years

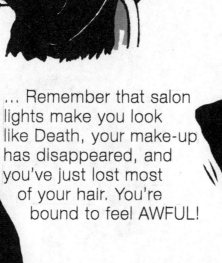

... Remember that salon lights make you look like Death, your make-up has disappeared, and you've just lost most of your hair. You're bound to feel AWFUL!

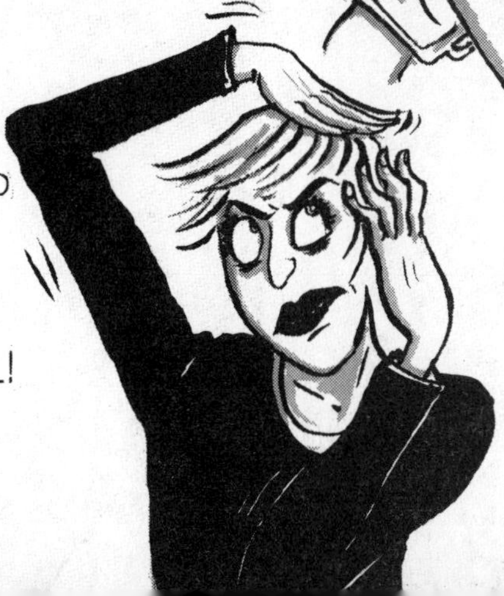

Play around with it for a while. You usually find it's not as bad as you first thought.

Every now and again someone has a haircut that ruins their life. They get a massive insecurity complex and have to get used to HATS.
So how can we possibly make sure we get the look we want?

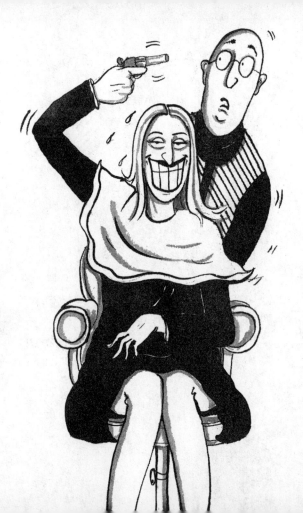

DIETS

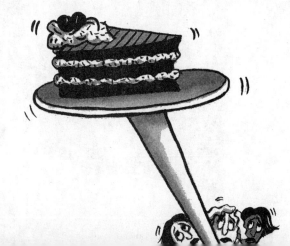

Diets are something we all seem to be on at one time
or other. Being larger than you'd like can take over
your life, and women really can bore you to death
about their size, their clothes and their eating habits.
You wish they'd just shut up and enjoy themselves.
That is, until you suddenly find you can't get into
your trousers and you drastically need to DIET!

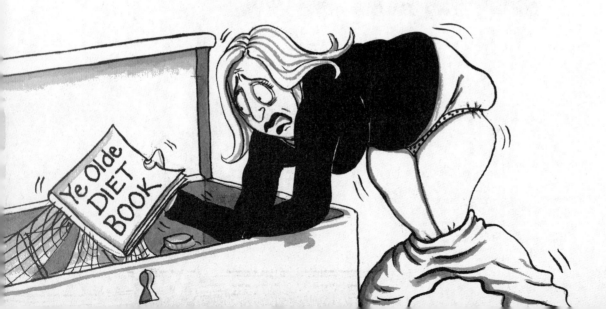

As soon as you start to Diet, you notice that you're completely surrounded by THIN PEOPLE.
Magazines are full of thin people, newspapers are full of thin people; there are posters of thin people everywhere ... and when you turn on the television, everyone's thin!

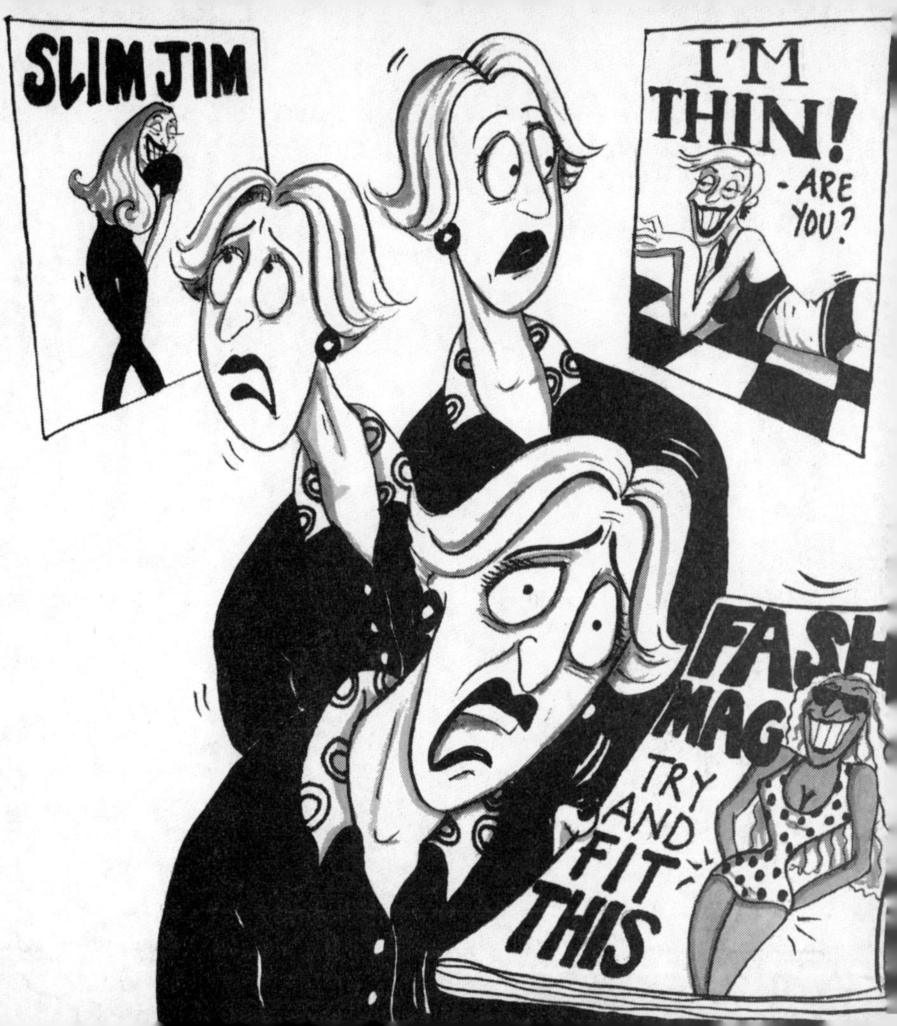
SLIM JIM
I'M THIN! - ARE YOU?
FASH MAG
TRY AND FIT THIS

So you begin to TORTURE yourself. You think about food all the time, when you *never* did before ...

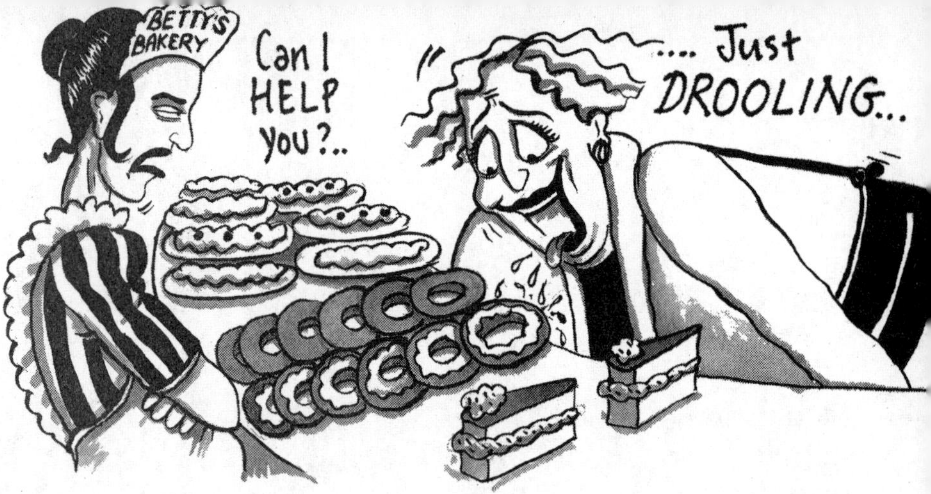
BETTY'S BAKERY
Can I HELP you?..
".... Just DROOLING...

... and you eventually end up *eating* more, mainly because you're forever rewarding yourself for not filling your face with everything in sight ...

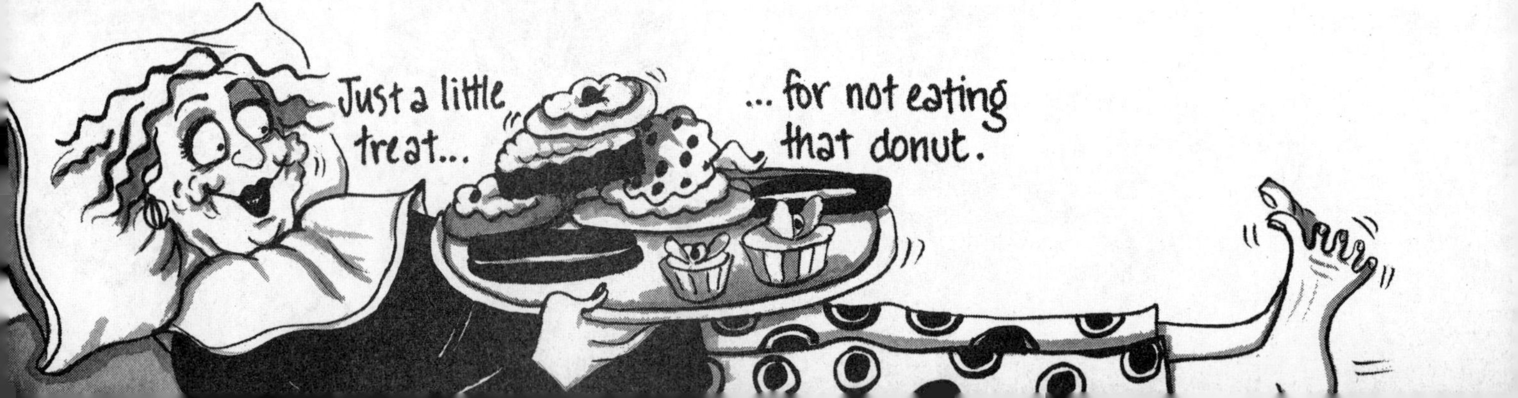
Just a little treat...
... for not eating that donut.

... You constantly look at other people's hips to see if they're smaller than yours, and to REALLY depress yourself, you get out the photo album and look at yourself when you were 15 ...

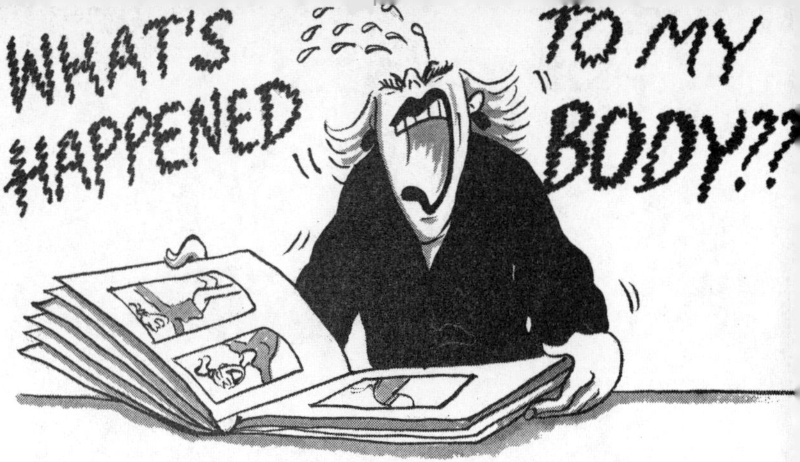
WHAT'S HAPPENED TO MY BODY??

... And you find yourself sneaking into OUTSIZE SHOPS, just to try on clothes that are guaranteed to be too big.

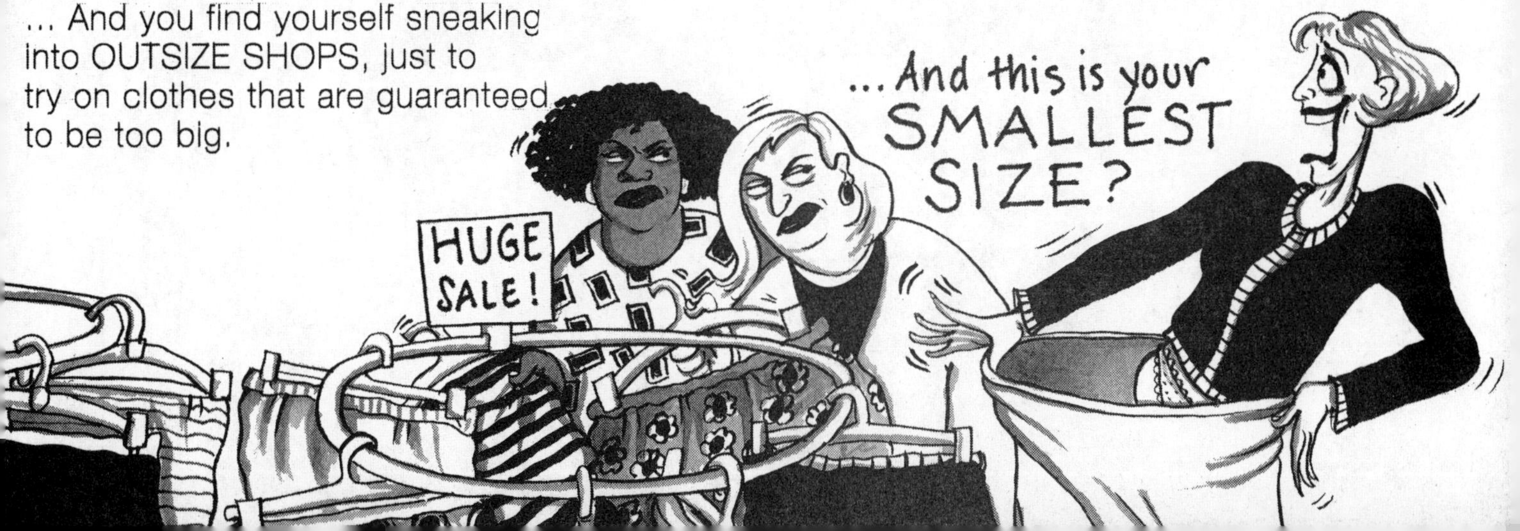
HUGE SALE!
...And this is your SMALLEST SIZE?

YOU KNOW YOU NEED TO DIET WHEN ...

... YOU stop moving ... but your bottom doesn't ...

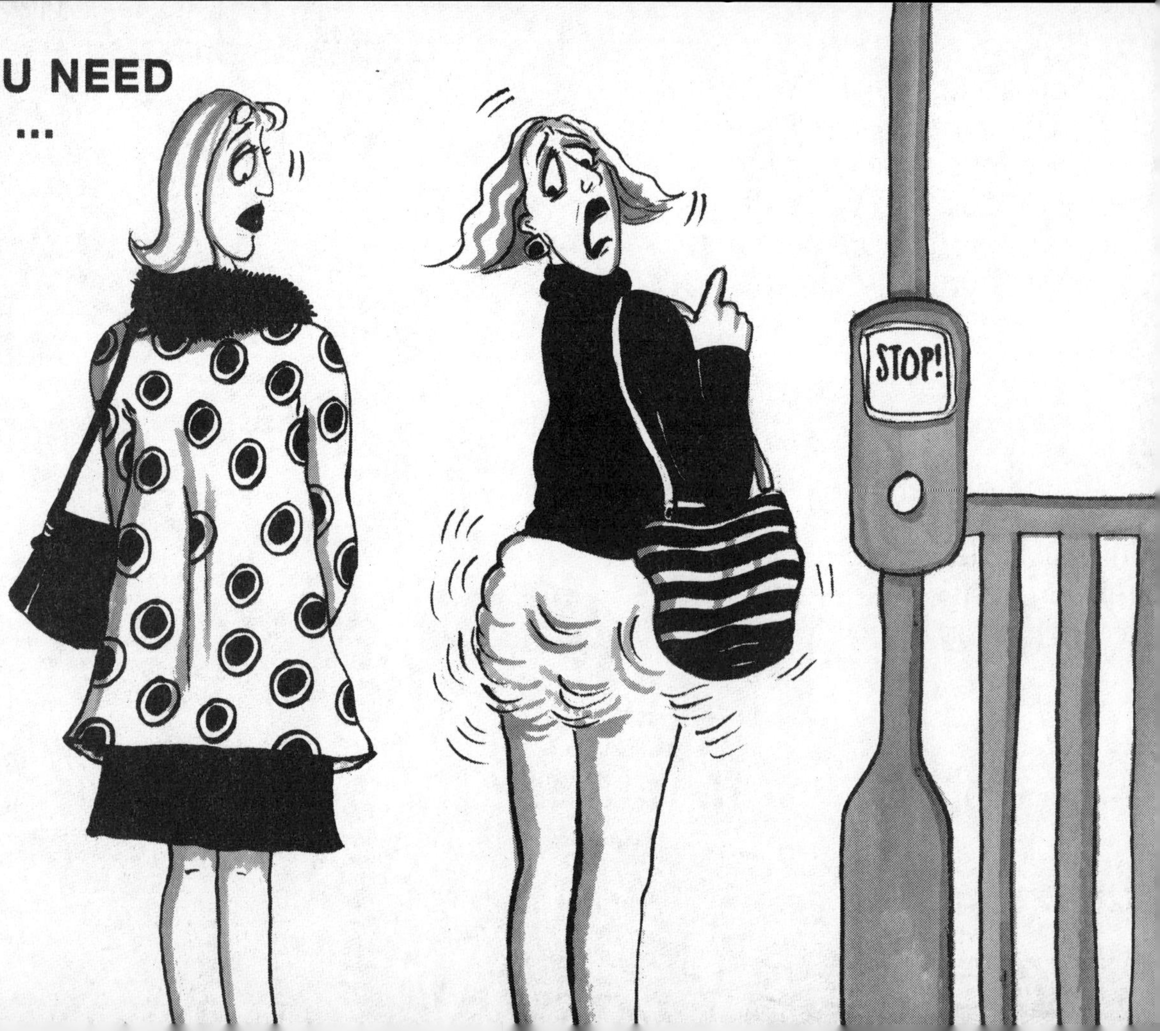
STOP!

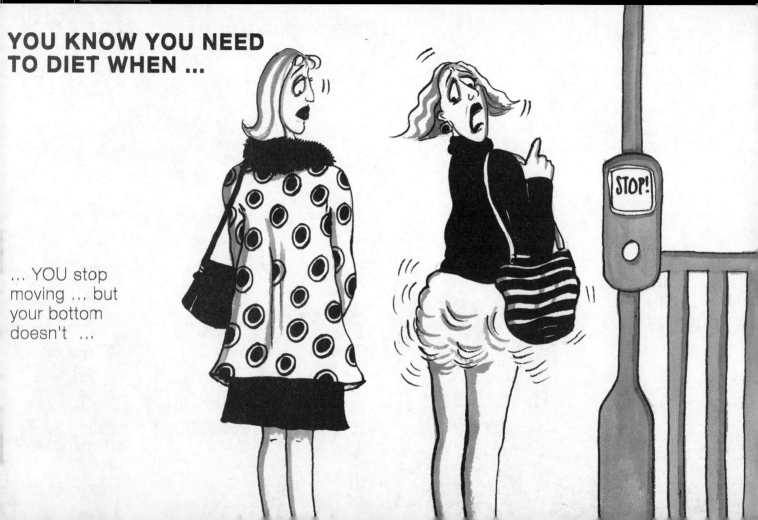

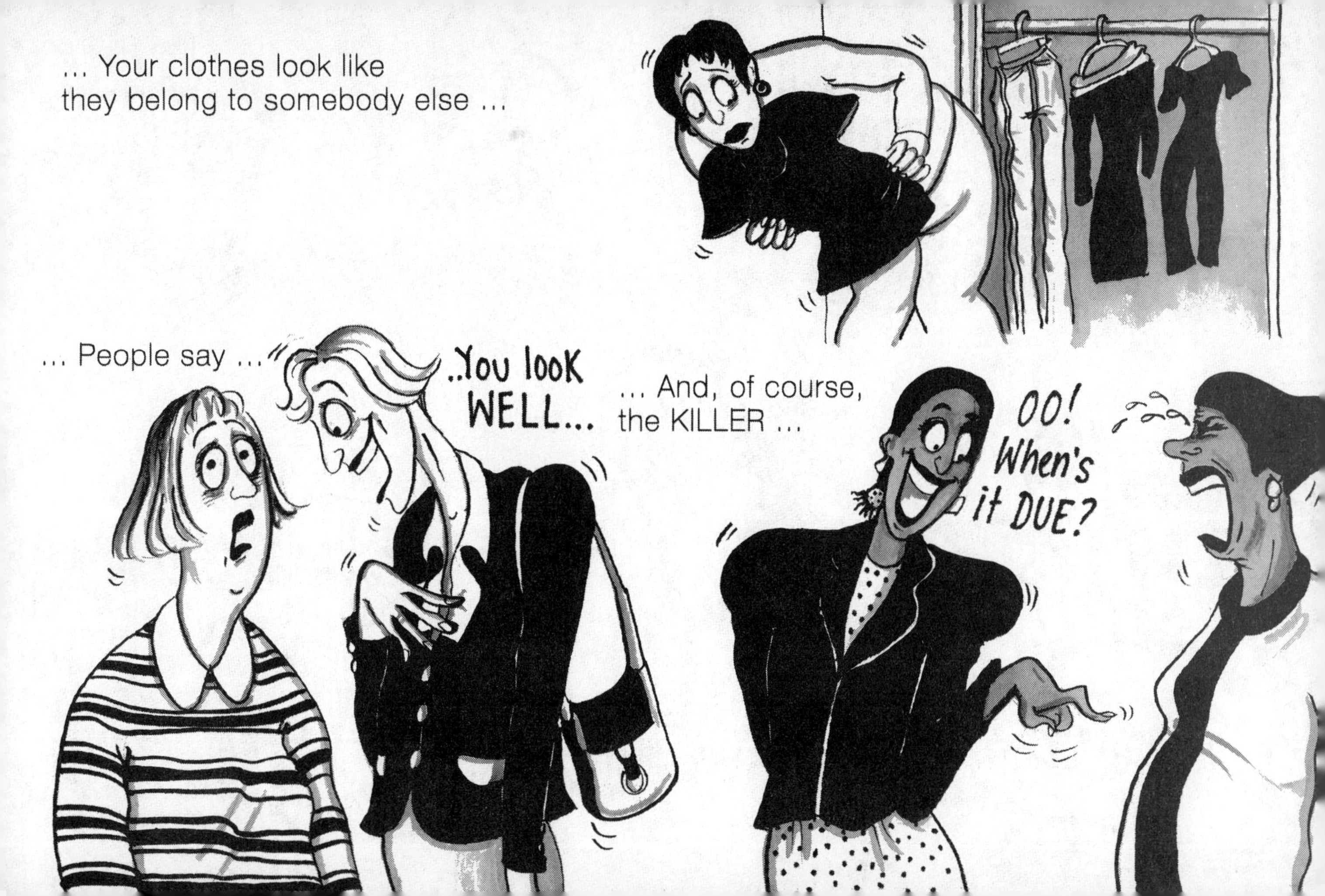
... Your clothes look like
they belong to somebody else ...
... People say ...
..You look
WELL...
... And, of course,
the KILLER ...
OO!
When's
it DUE?

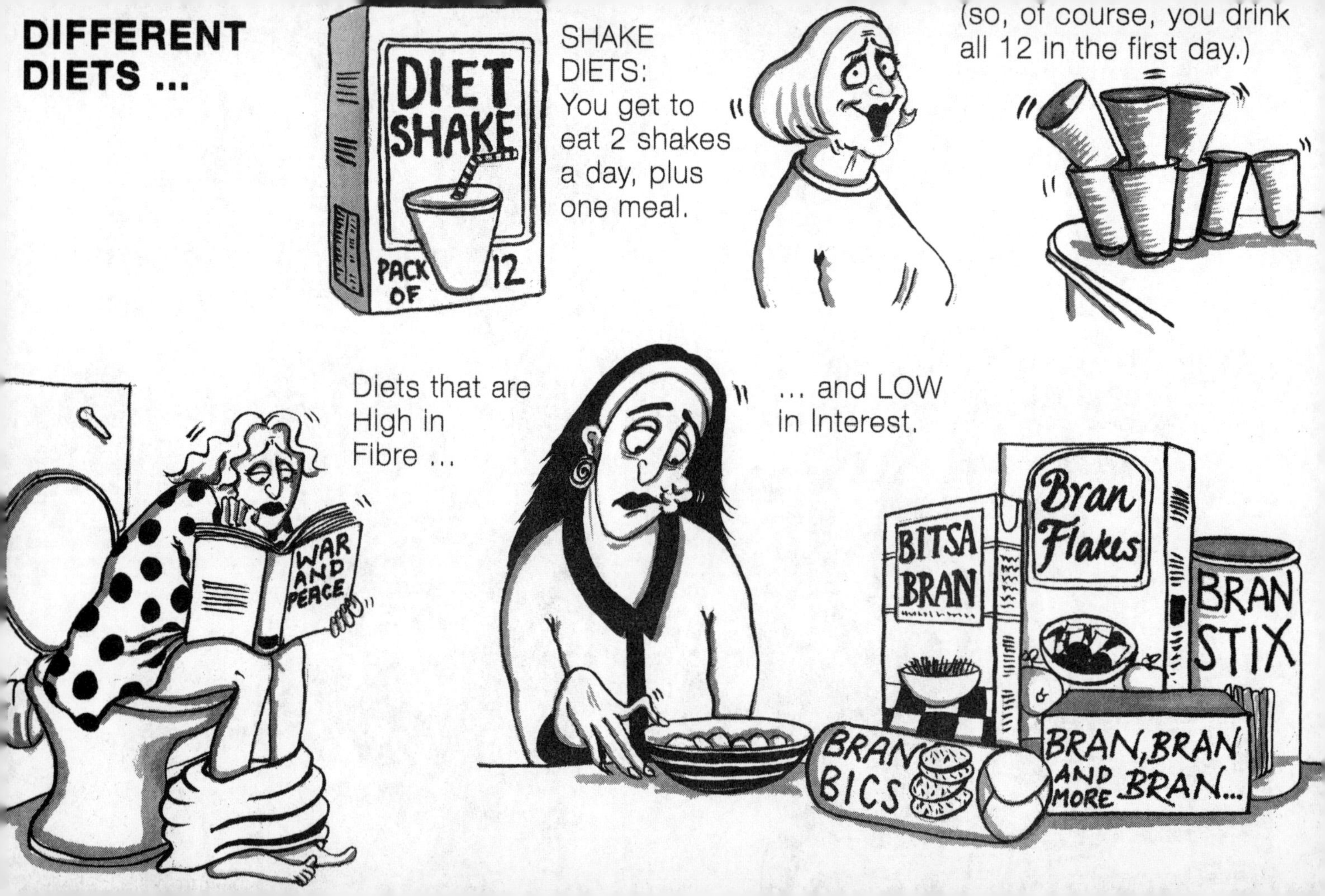
DIFFERENT DIETS ...
DIET SHAKE
PACK OF 12
SHAKE DIETS: You get to eat 2 shakes a day, plus one meal.
(so, of course, you drink all 12 in the first day.)
Diets that are High in Fibre ...
... and LOW in Interest.
WAR AND PEACE
BITSA BRAN
Bran Flakes
BRAN STIX
BRAN BICS
BRAN, BRAN AND MORE BRAN...

The "Eat As Much As You Can And Then Throw Up Afterwards" Diet ...

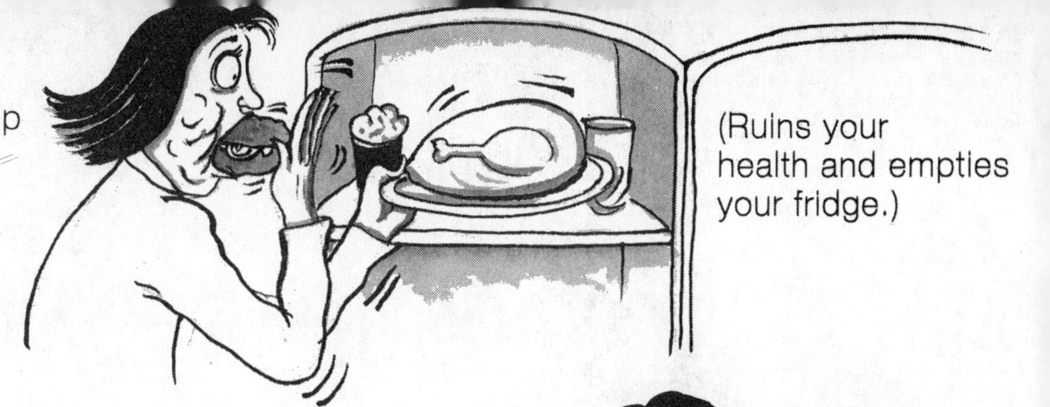

(Ruins your health and empties your fridge.)

Hypnosis ... or self hypnosis ...

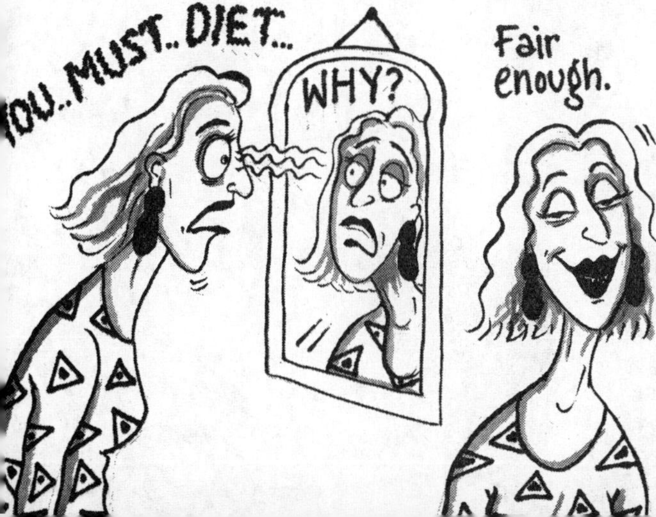
OU..MUST..DIET...
WHY?
Fair enough.

... and if you're particularly weak, Slim-As-You-Sleep cassettes you listen to at night.

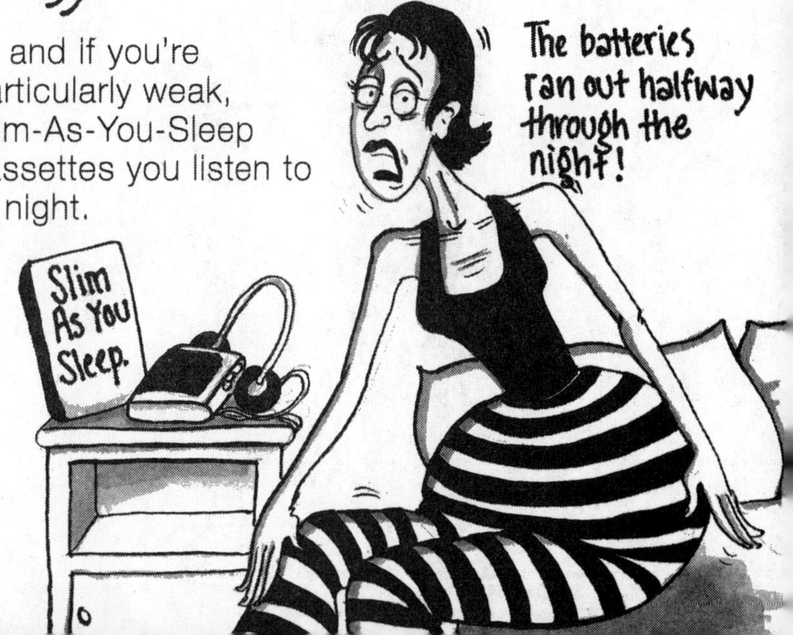
Slim As You Sleep.
The batteries ran out halfway through the night!

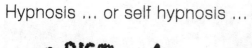

Sometimes you can manage to control your willpower and stick to diets for months at a time.

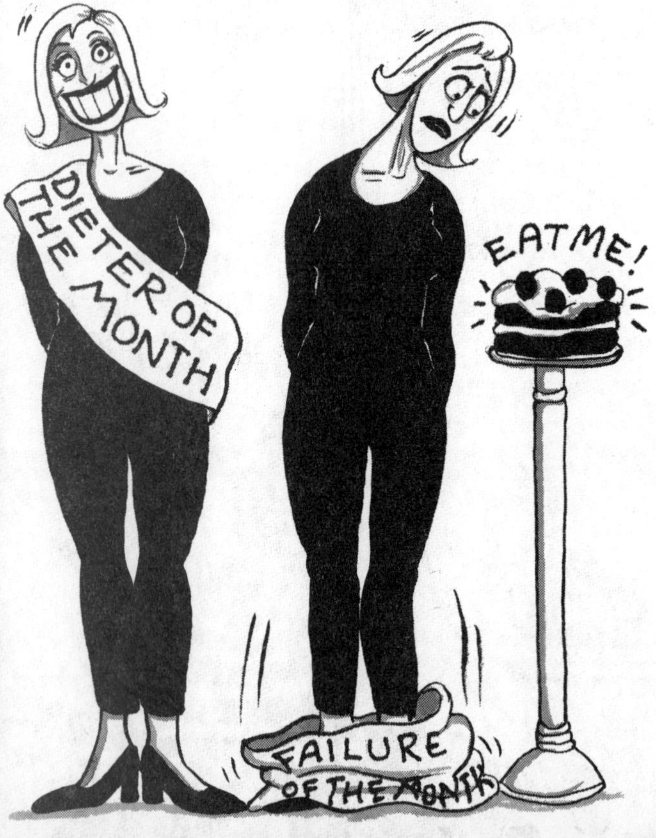
DIETER OF THE MONTH
EAT ME!
FAILURE OF THE MONTH

But you can *guarantee* that as soon as you have a relapse and settle down in front of the television for a good old stuff, someone skinny will appear leaping about in a leotard. You just can't win.

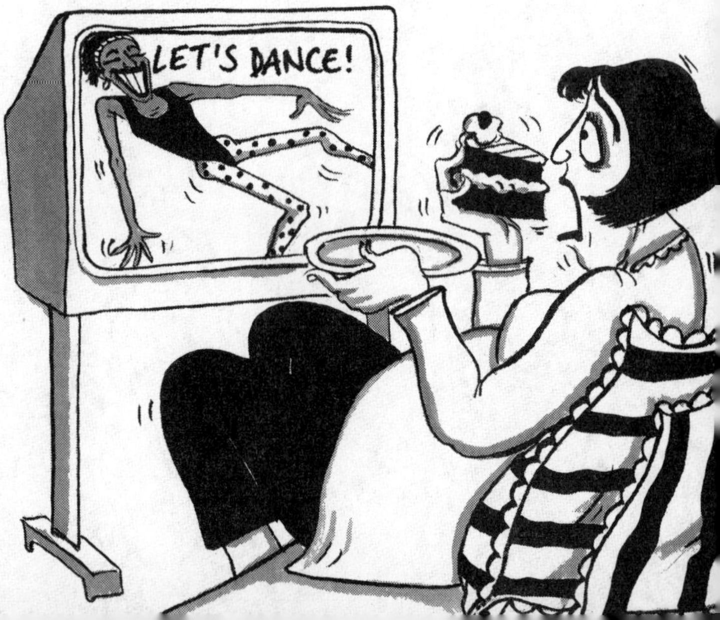
LET'S DANCE!

The greatest pressure when you're dieting is that you may turn into a DIET BORE. Fascinating though it may be to you, other people aren't interested in your daily calorie intake, the workings of your digestive juices, and how much weight you've lost in the past minute and a half.

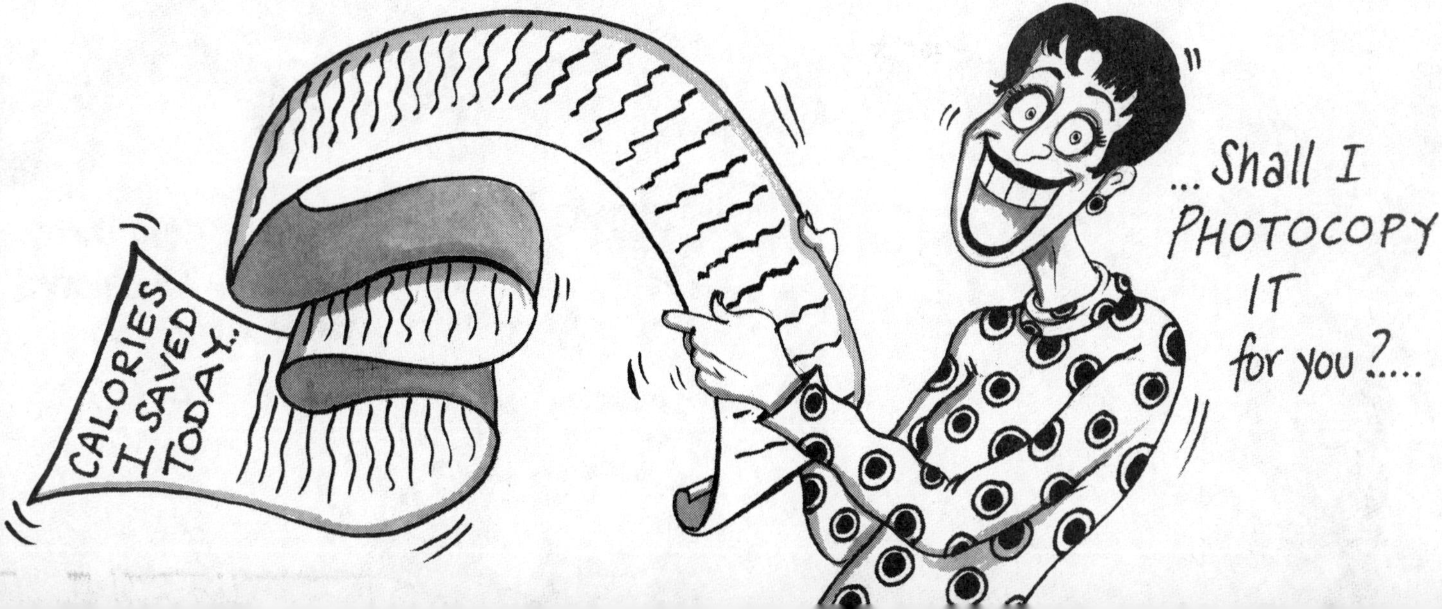
CALORIES I SAVED TODAY..
...Shall I PHOTOCOPY IT for you?....

HOW TO SPOT A DIET BORE ...

There are Diet Bores who skip their lunch and spend their time dribbling over yours; Bores who did biology at school and go into gruesome detail of how each meal is broken down ... and then there are the slim, attractive women who just go on and on ...

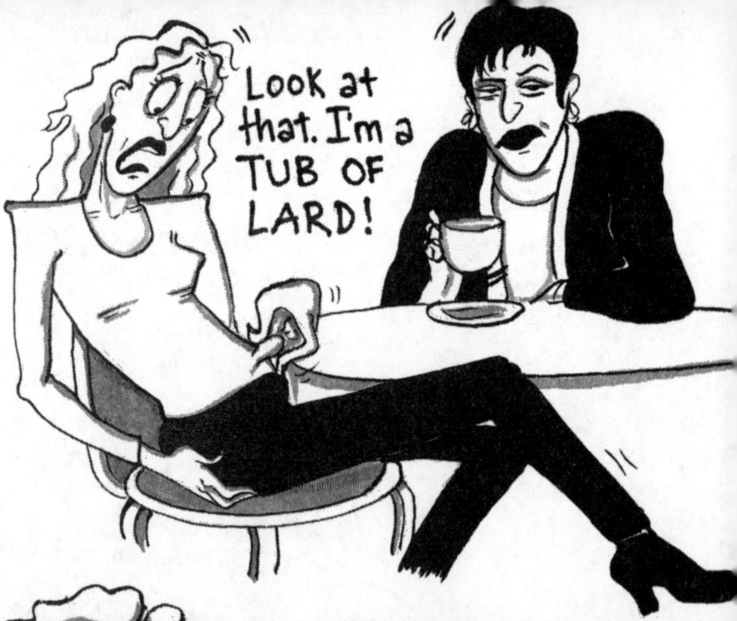
Look at that. I'm a TUB OF LARD!

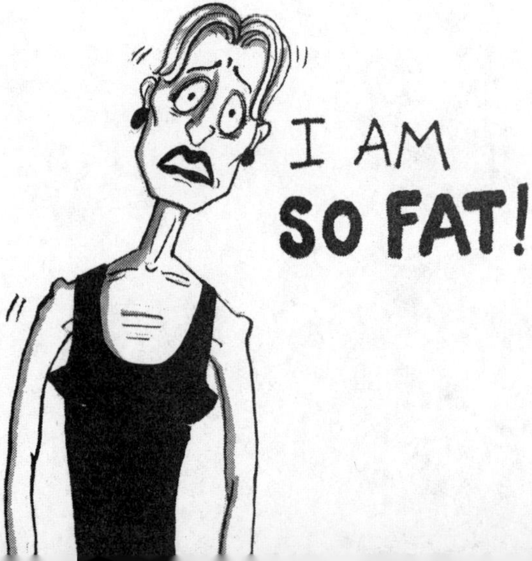
I AM SO FAT!

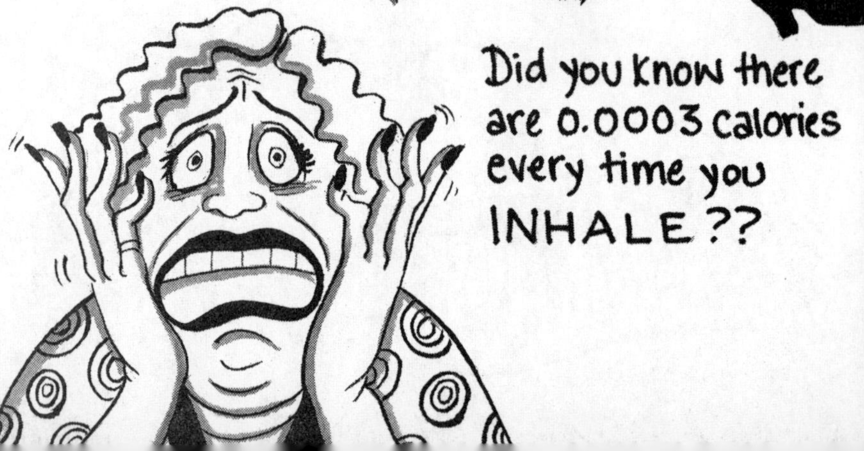
Did you know there are 0.0003 calories every time you INHALE ??

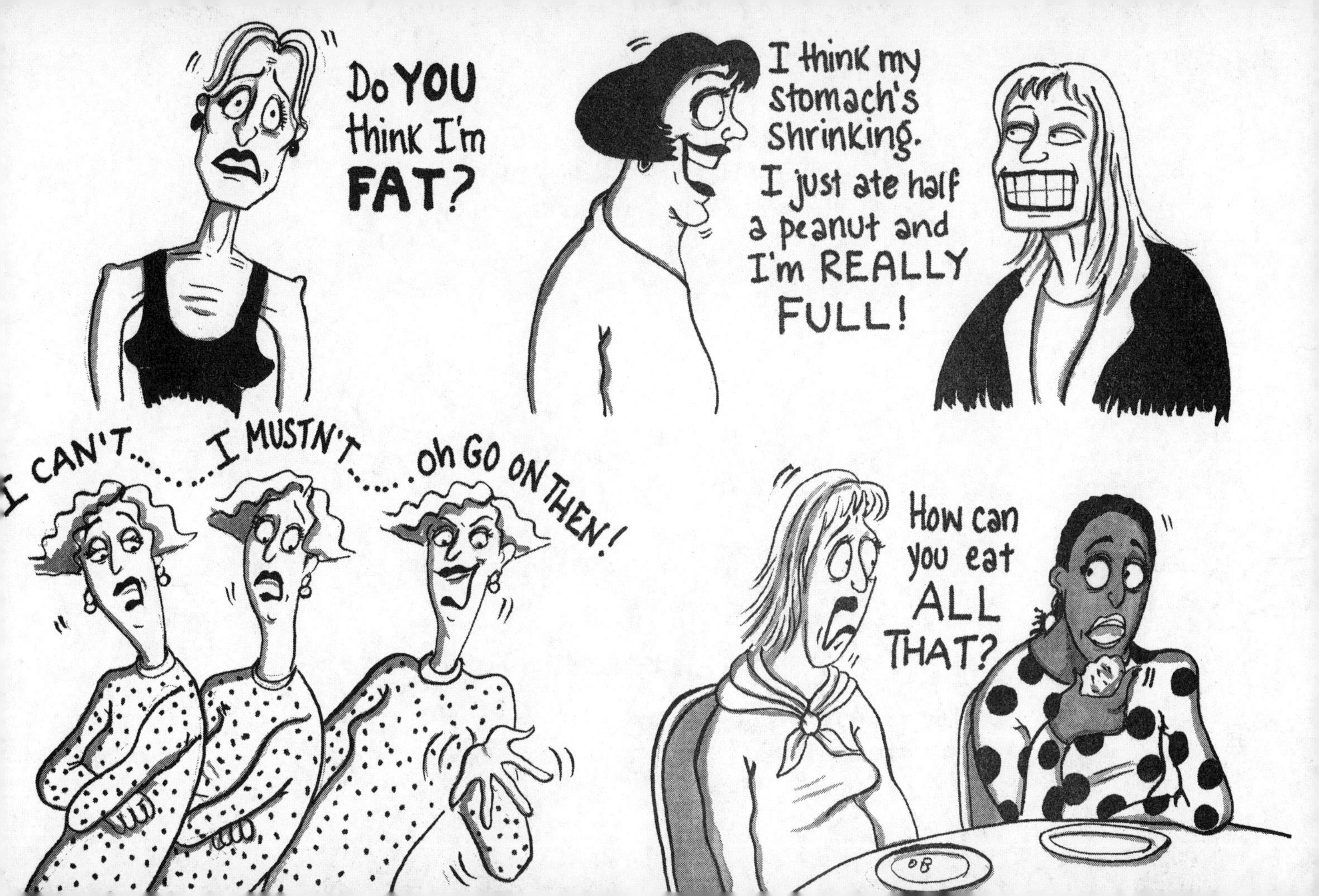
Do YOU think I'm FAT?
I think my stomach's shrinking. I just ate half a peanut and I'm REALLY FULL!
I CAN'T..... I MUSTN'T...... oh GO ON THEN!
How can you eat ALL THAT?

Being FAT makes you miserable, DIETING makes you miserable; you spend twice the money eating half as much, you're HELL to know ... so is it really WORTH IT?

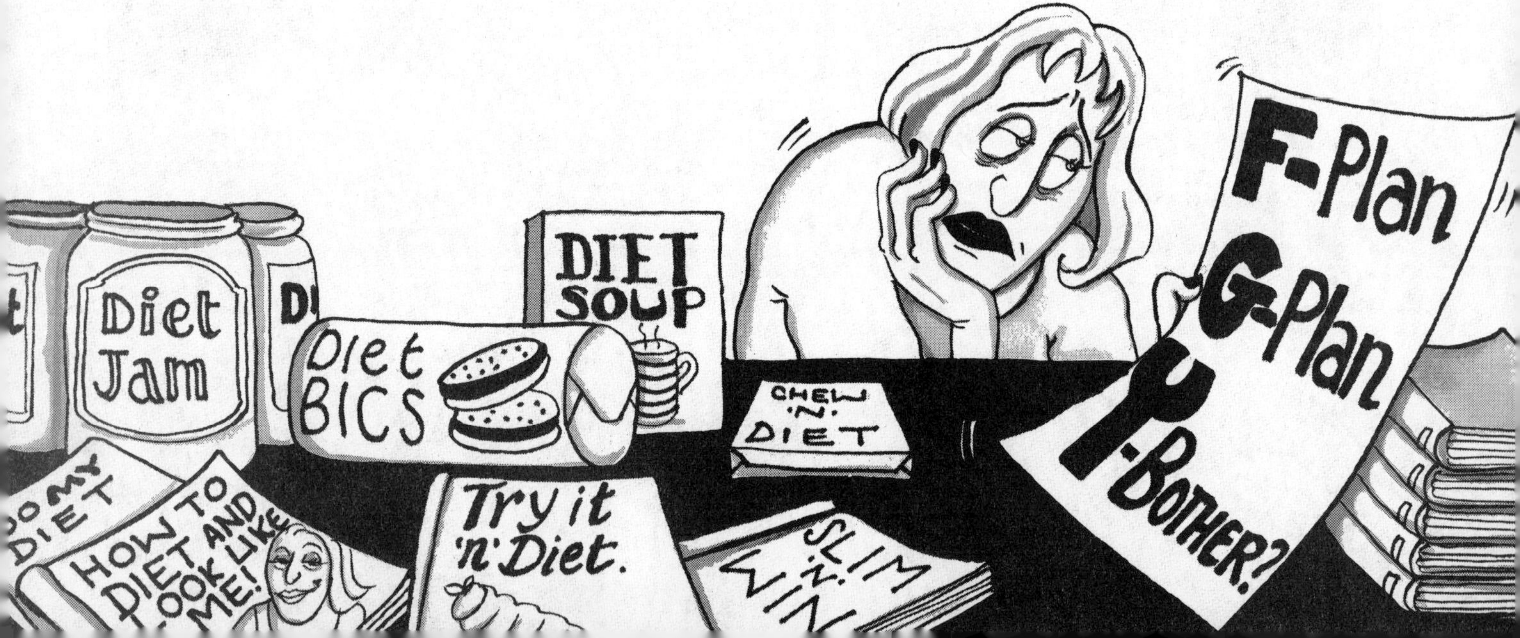

Diet Jam
DIET SOUP
Diet BICS
CHEW 'N' DIET
F-Plan
G-Plan
Y-Bother?
Try it 'n' Diet.
HOW TO DIET AND LOOK LIKE ME!

EXERCISE

Step 3
NOW
P.T.O

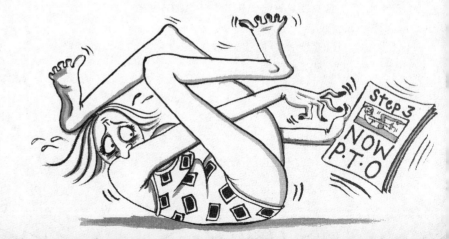

If we believed all that we read in magazines and newspapers, we'd never eat anything more than two crispbreads and a tomato pip and would be so thin we'd fall down the cracks in the pavement. The trend seems to be ever pushing towards the Exercised Body; when simple pleasures like donut-stuffing and staying in bed until 3 o'clock become cardinal sins; and admitting that you don't actually WANT to *Feel That Burn* can turn you into a social leper!

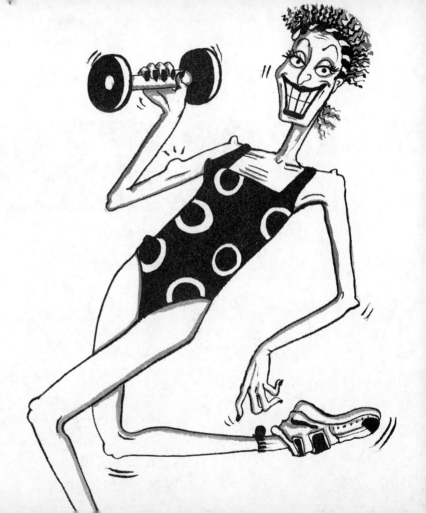

Some people can't just exercise a couple of times a week. Once they start, they quickly become addicted; it takes over their lives and they are completely OBSESSED.

They clench their buttocks all day at work.

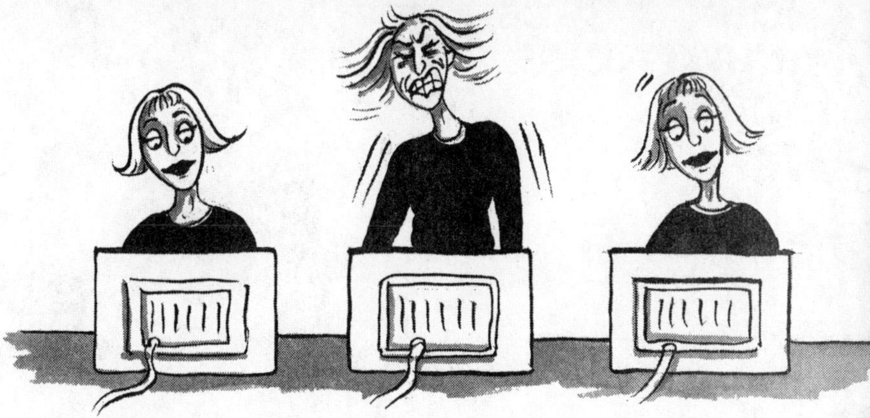

They can't stand still at Bus Stops.

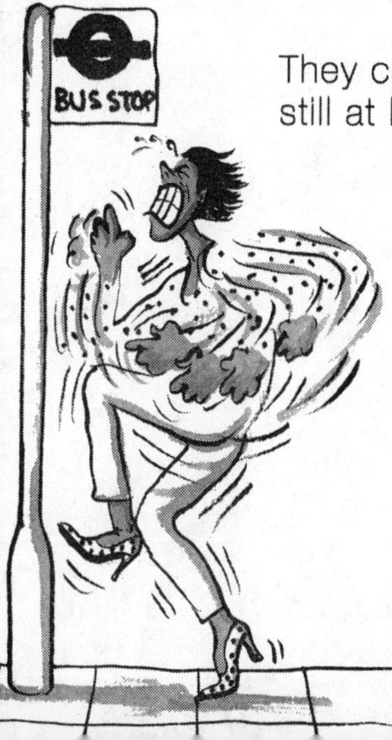
BUS STOP

They don't let themselves relax for a moment.

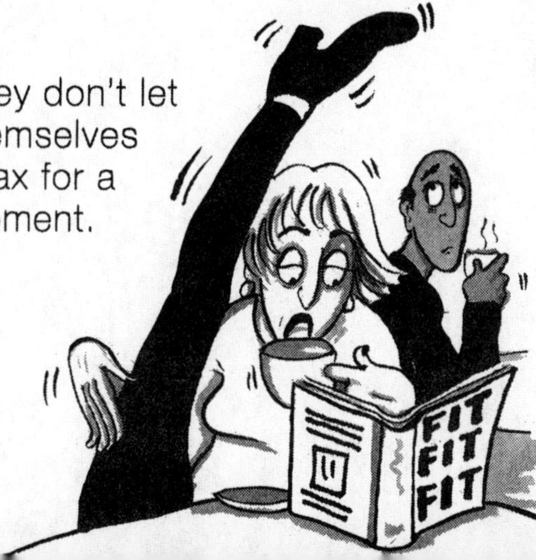
FIT
FIT
FIT

... and if they're not careful, they turn into an EXERCISE BORE.

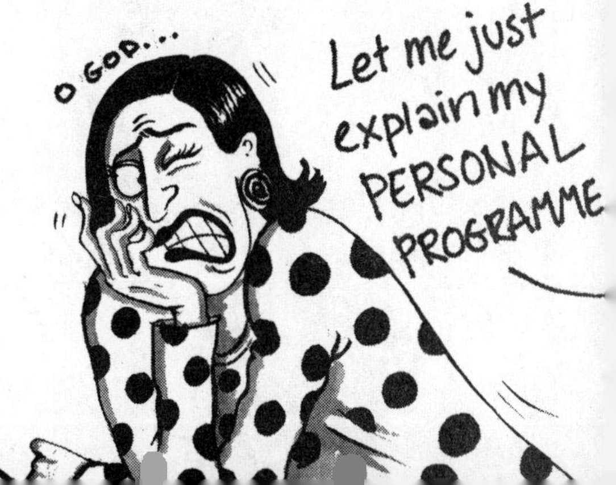
O GOD...
Let me just explain my PERSONAL PROGRAMME

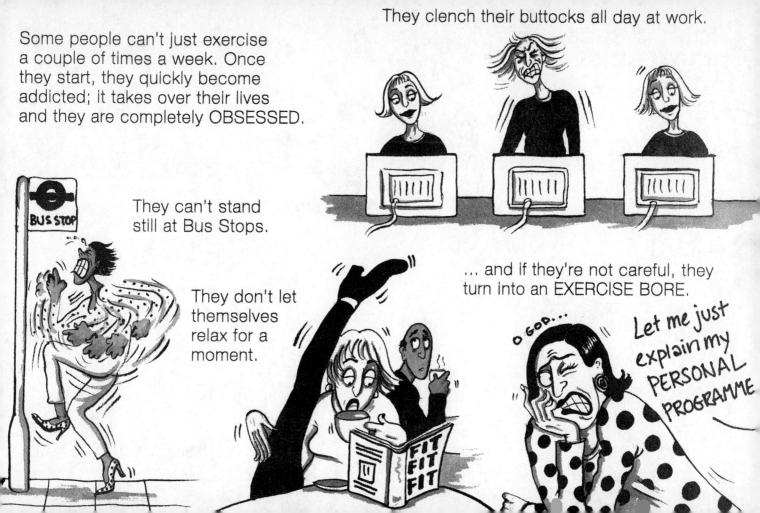

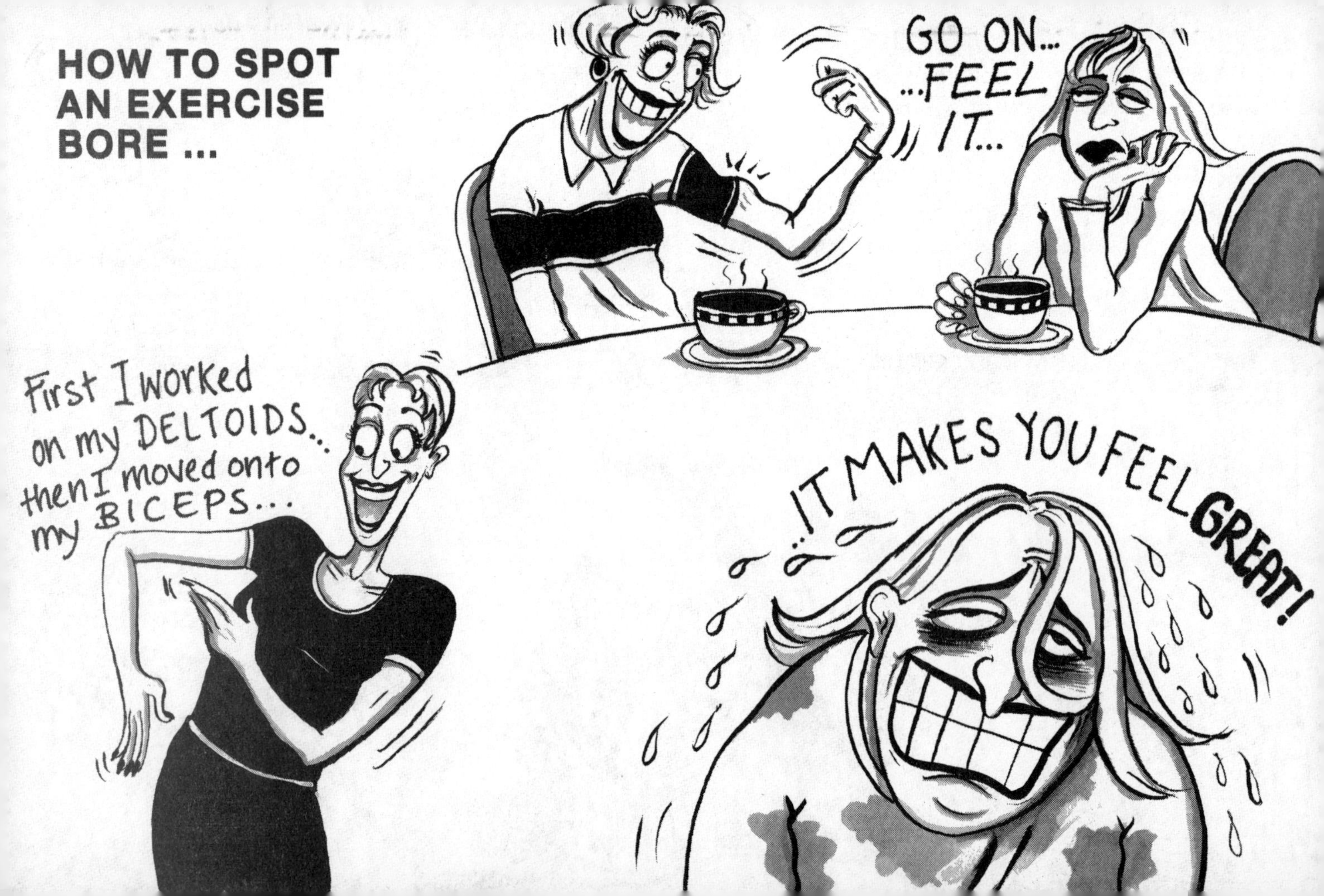
HOW TO SPOT AN EXERCISE BORE ...
GO ON... ...FEEL IT...
First I worked on my DELTOIDS... then I moved onto my BICEPS...
...IT MAKES YOU FEEL GREAT!

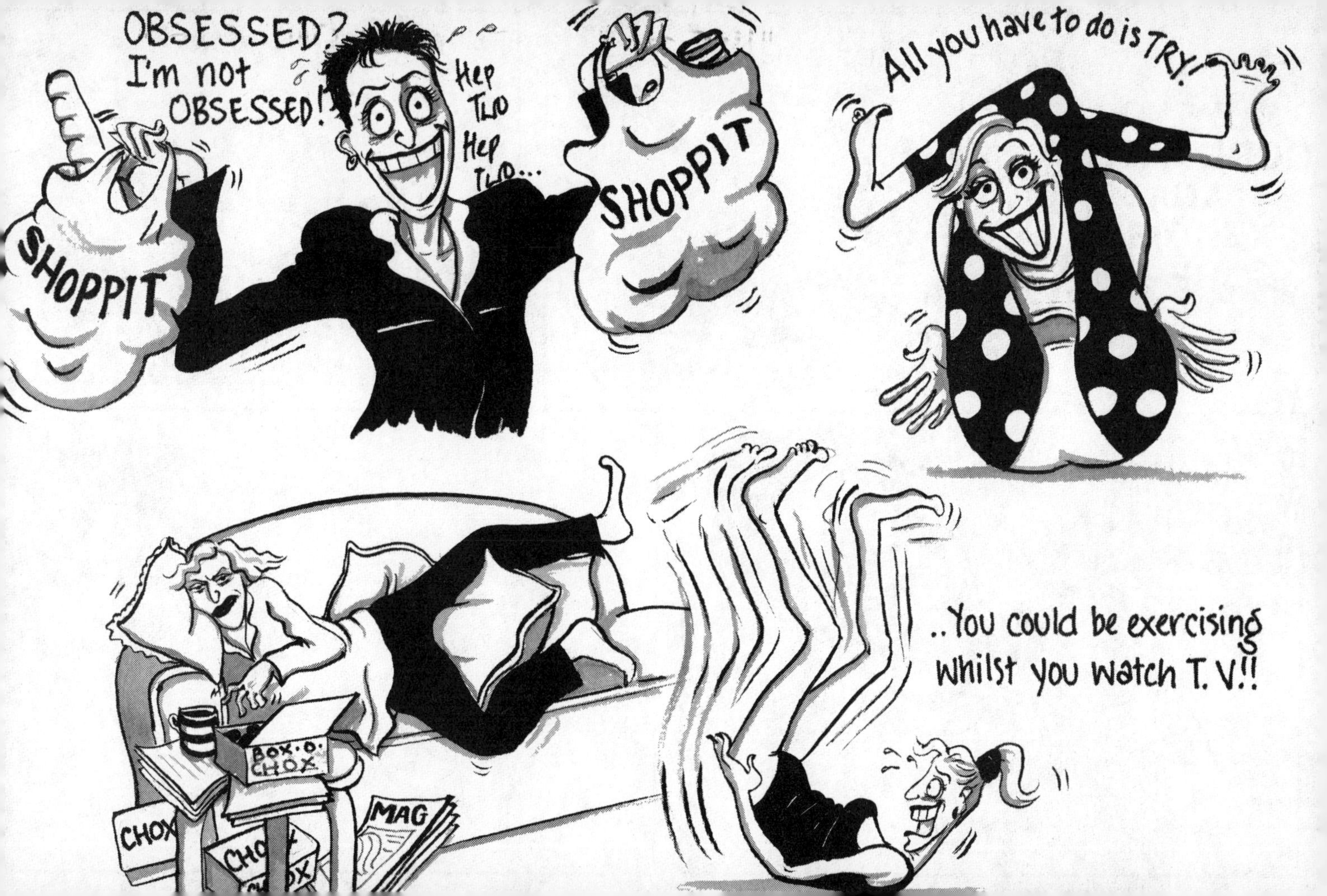
OBSESSED? I'm not OBSESSED!
Hep Two Hep Two...
SHOPPIT
SHOPPIT
All you have to do is TRY.
BOX.O. CHOX
CHOX
MAG
..You could be exercising whilst you watch T.V!!

HOW TO COPE WITH AN EXERCISE BORE ...

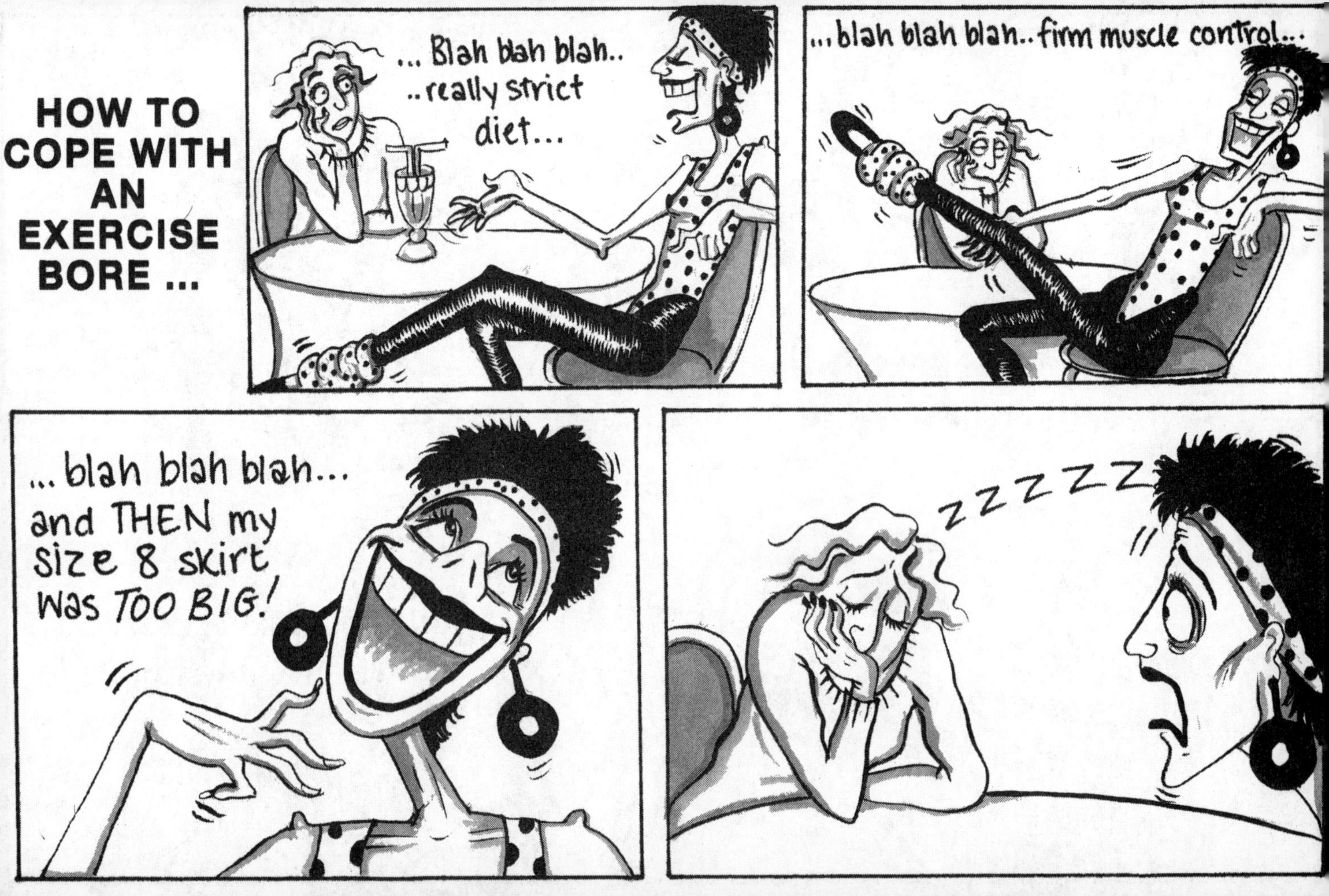
... Blah blah blah.. ..really strict diet...
...blah blah blah.. firm muscle control...
...blah blah blah... and THEN my size 8 skirt was TOO BIG!
ZZZZZZ

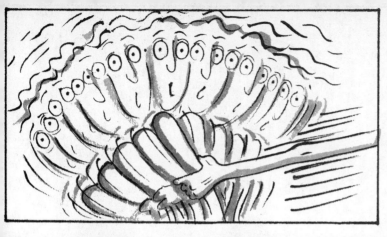

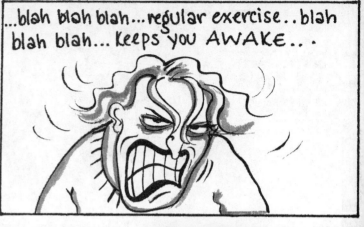

...blah blah blah...regular exercise..blah blah blah... Keeps you AWAKE...

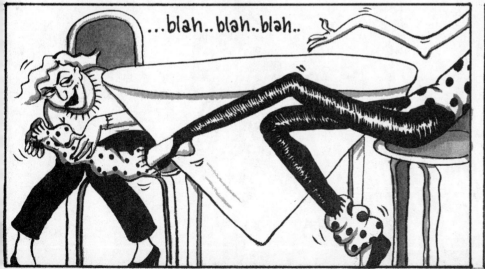

...blah..blah..blah..

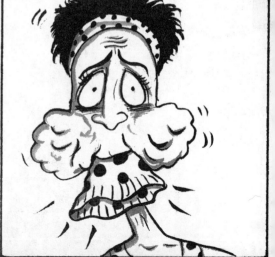

EASY WAYS TO EXERCISE

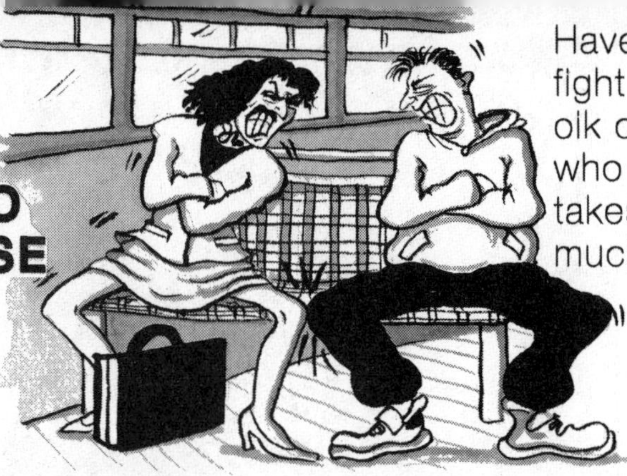

Have a daily fight with the oik on the bus who always takes up too much room ...

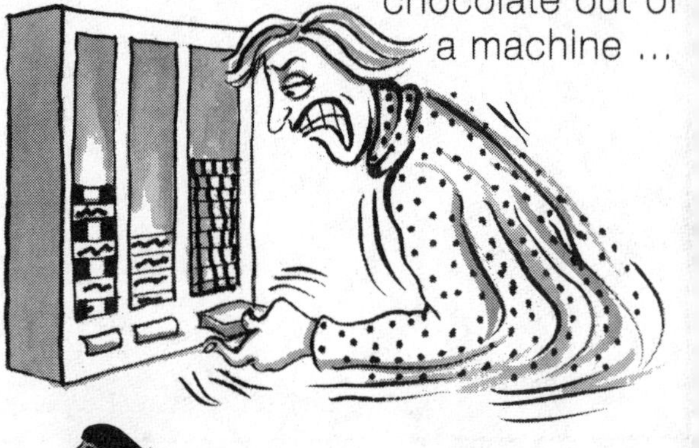

... Try and get chocolate out of a machine ...

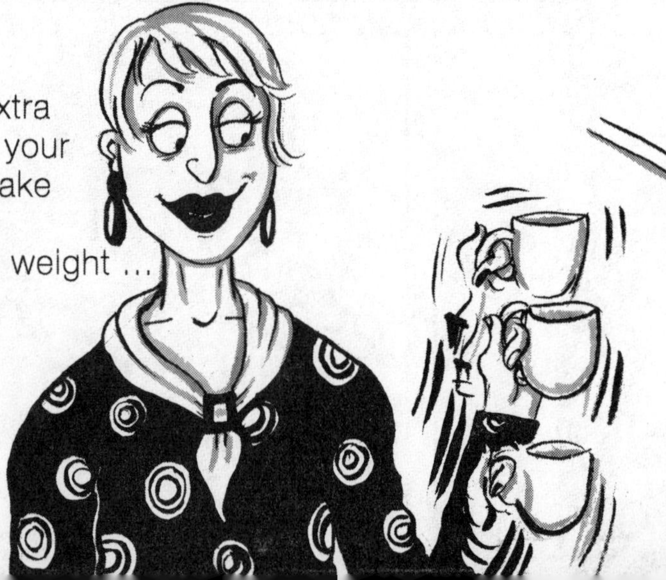

... Put extra sugar in your tea to make a more effective weight ...

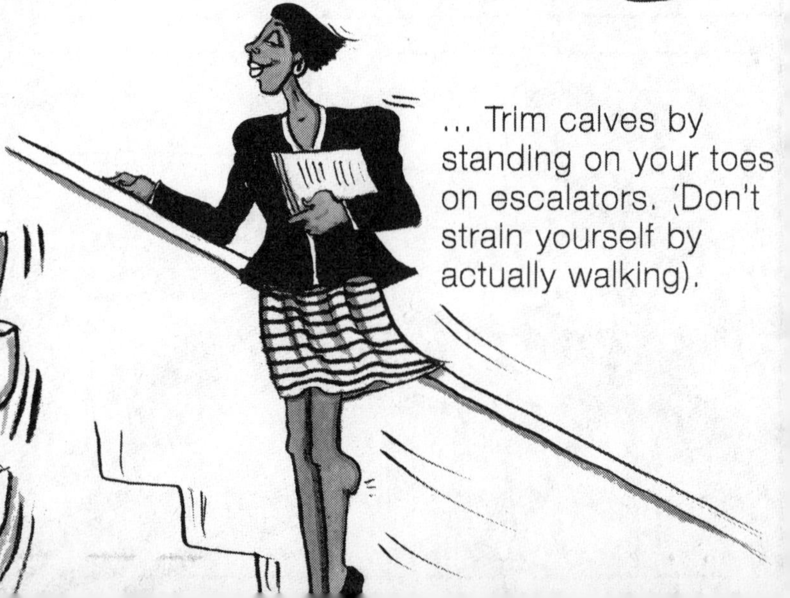

... Trim calves by standing on your toes on escalators. (Don't strain yourself by actually walking).

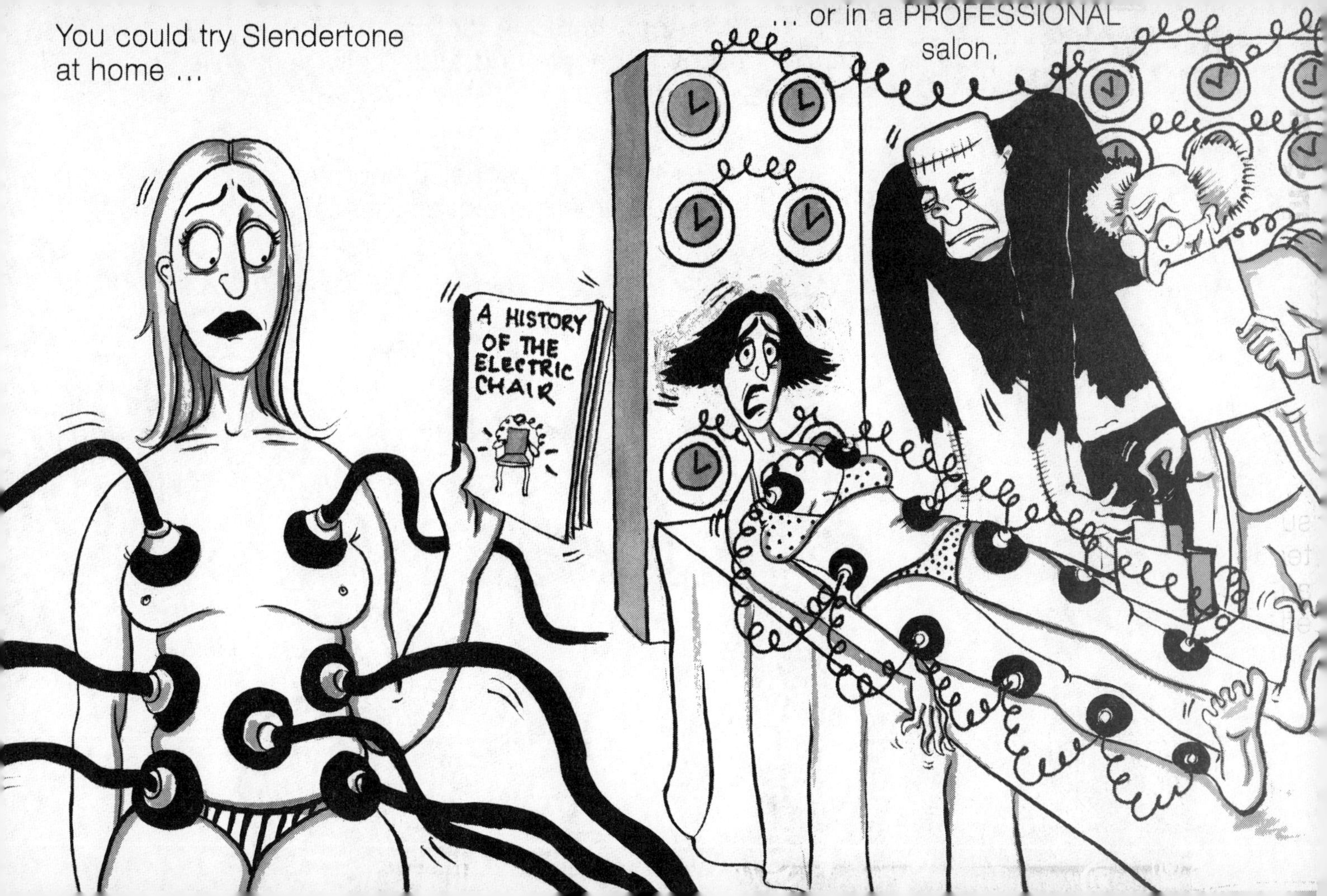
You could try Slendertone at home ...
... or in a PROFESSIONAL salon.
A HISTORY OF THE ELECTRIC CHAIR

HARD WAYS TO EXERCISE ...

Join a GYM. Apart from the fact that you're surrounded by fit people and feel totally demoralised; ... it *Really Hurts.*

You're given a Personal Trainer who puts you through a gruelling exercise session ...

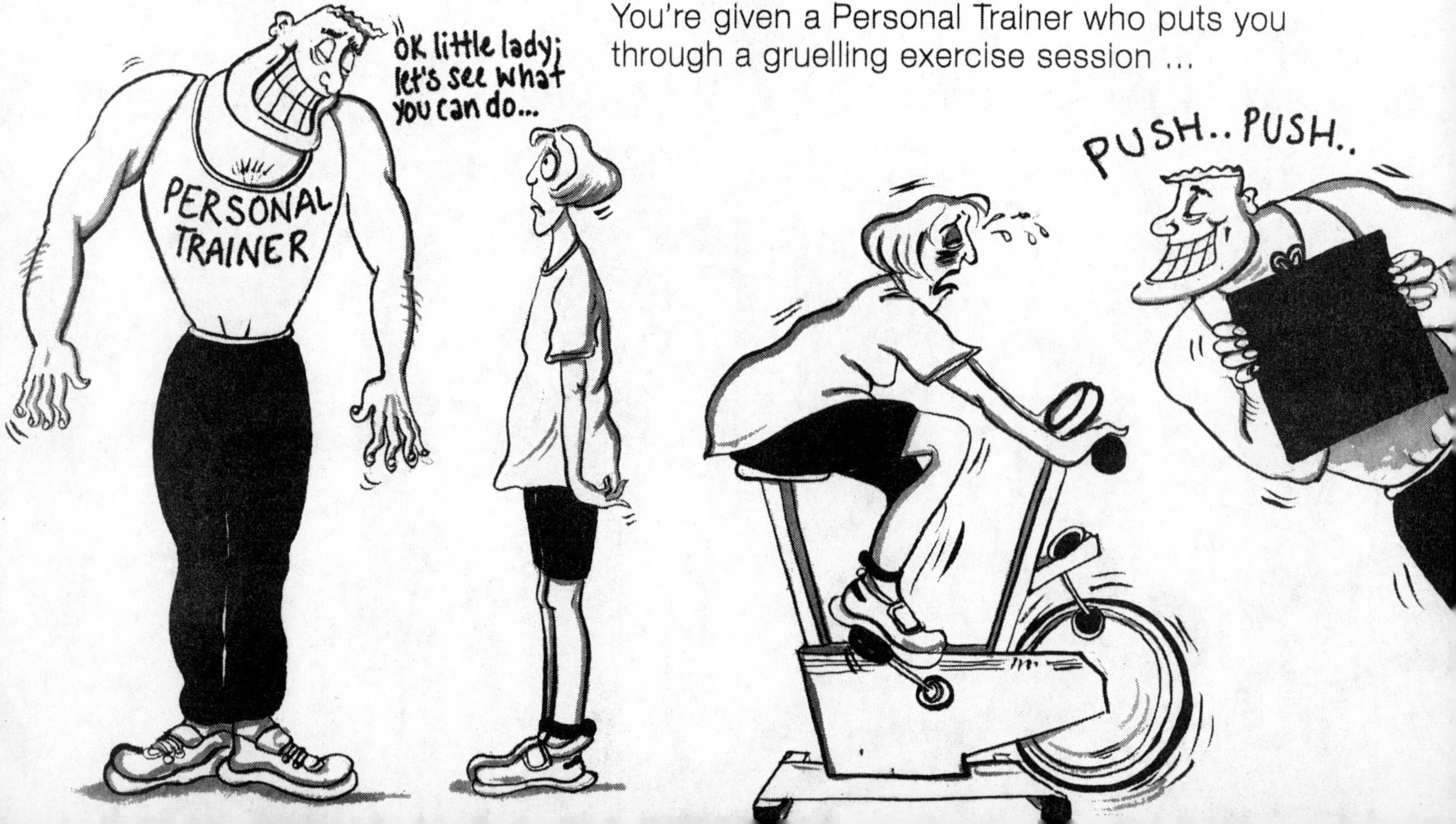
OK little lady; let's see what you can do...
PERSONAL TRAINER
PUSH.. PUSH..

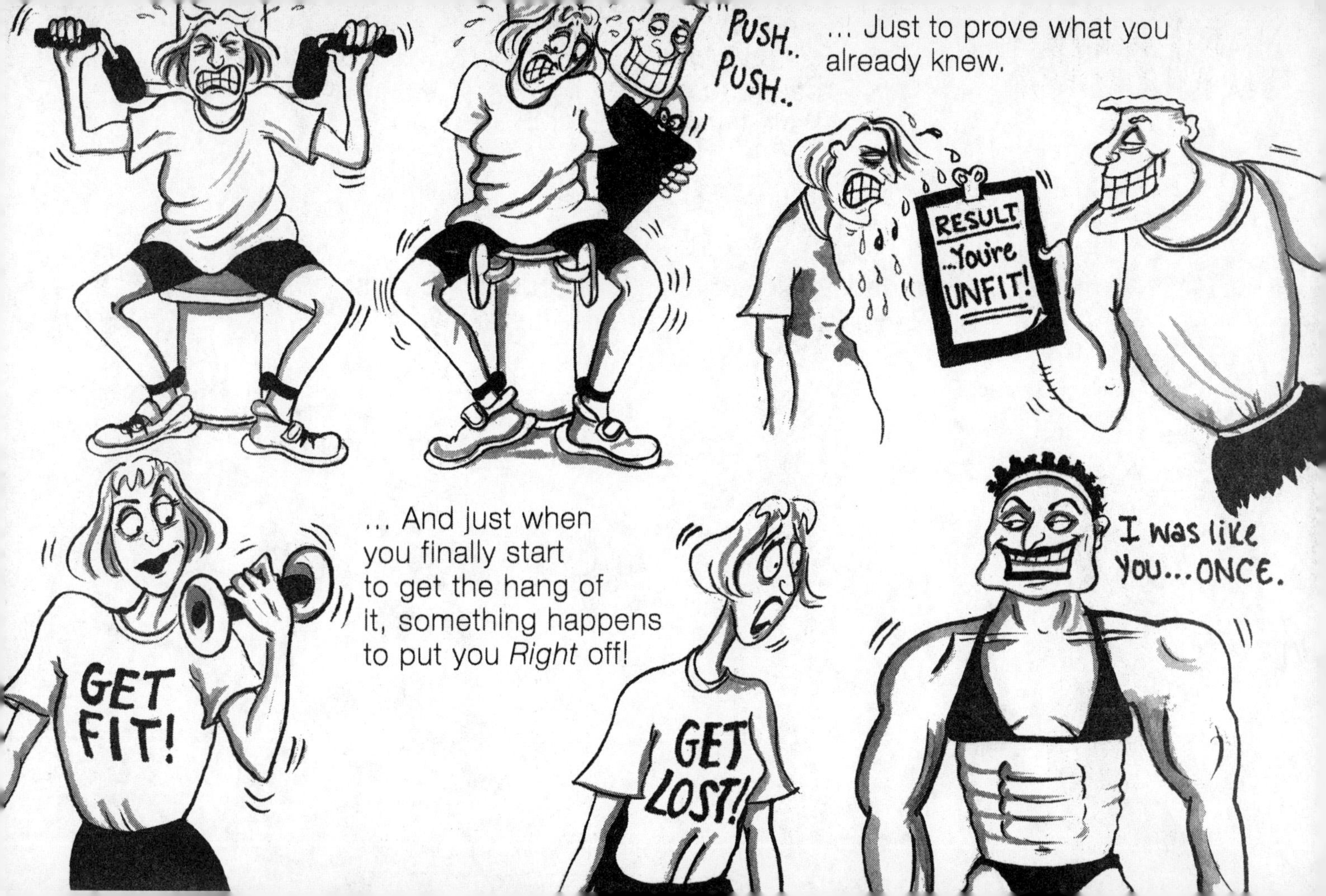
PUSH..
PUSH..
... Just to prove what you already knew.
RESULT
...You're UNFIT!
GET FIT!
... And just when you finally start to get the hang of it, something happens to put you *Right* off!
GET LOST!
I was like you...ONCE.

... or you could try SWIMMING.

It's a vicious circle .. you go swimming so you can tone up your body ... but in order to swim you have to wear a SWIMSUIT.

How can you endure looking at this year's body in last year's smimsuit?

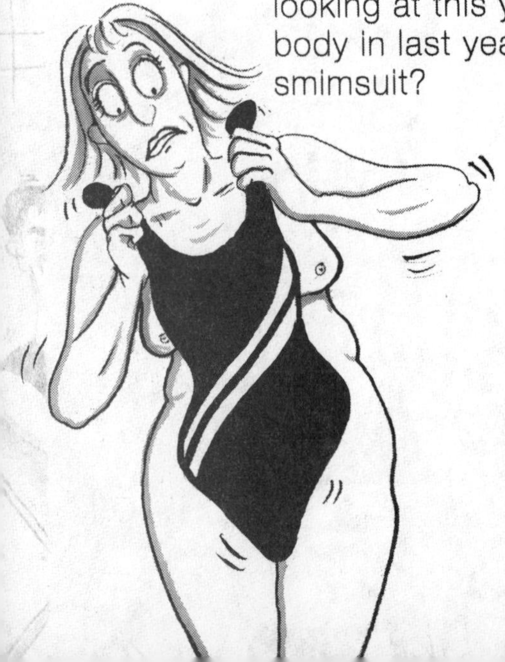

... You don't! You just refuse to take your TOWEL OFF!

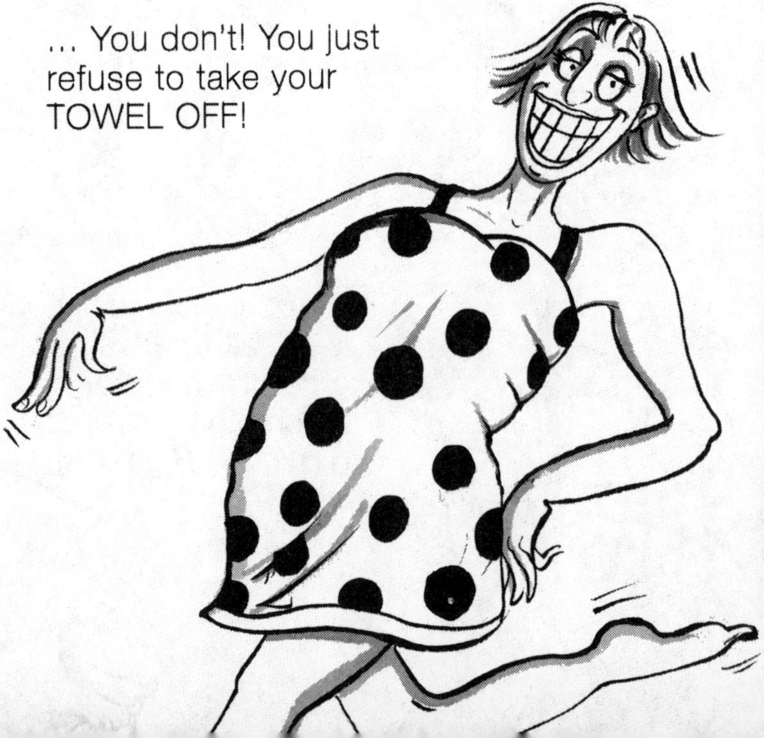

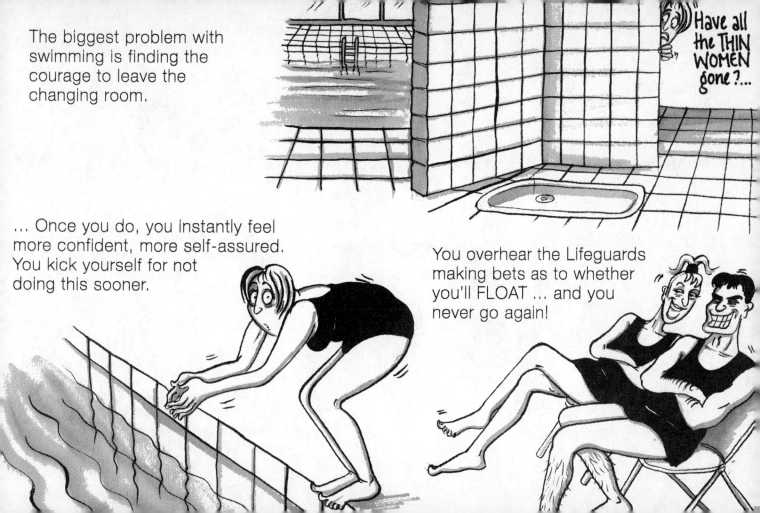

The biggest problem with swimming is finding the courage to leave the changing room.

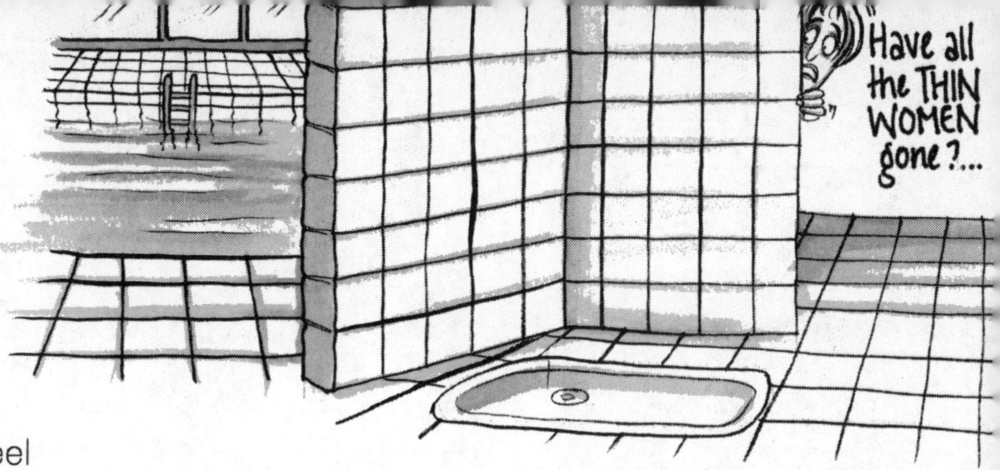
"Have all the THIN WOMEN gone?..."

... Once you do, you instantly feel more confident, more self-assured. You kick yourself for not doing this sooner.

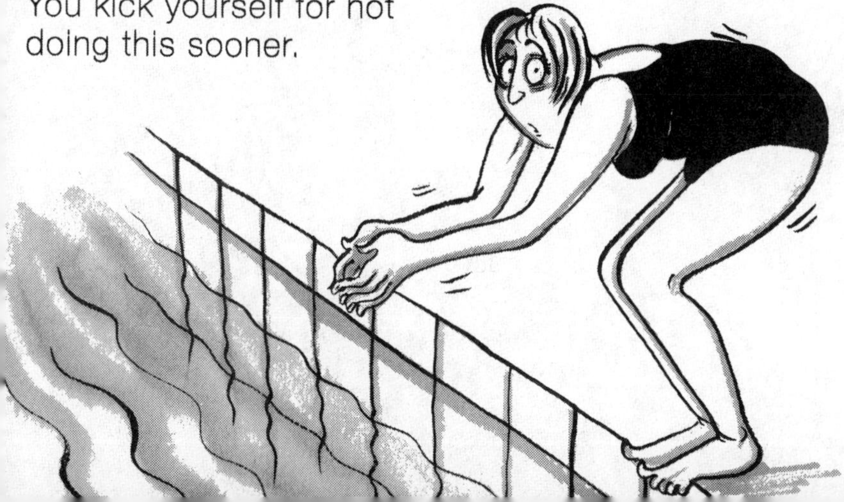

You overhear the Lifeguards making bets as to whether you'll FLOAT ... and you never go again!

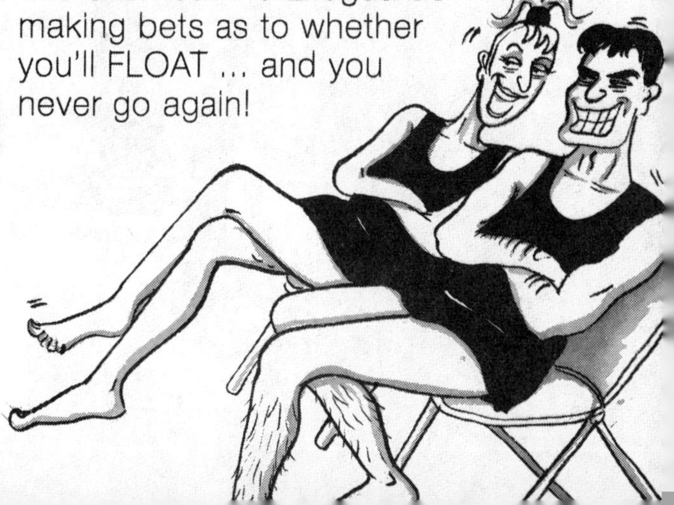

You could buy one of the hundreds of VIDEOS available and exercise in your own home.

The ADVANTAGES are that no-one can see you wobble, go red, or hear you grunt.

The DISADVANTAGES are finding a convenient time ... and finding your WILL POWER.

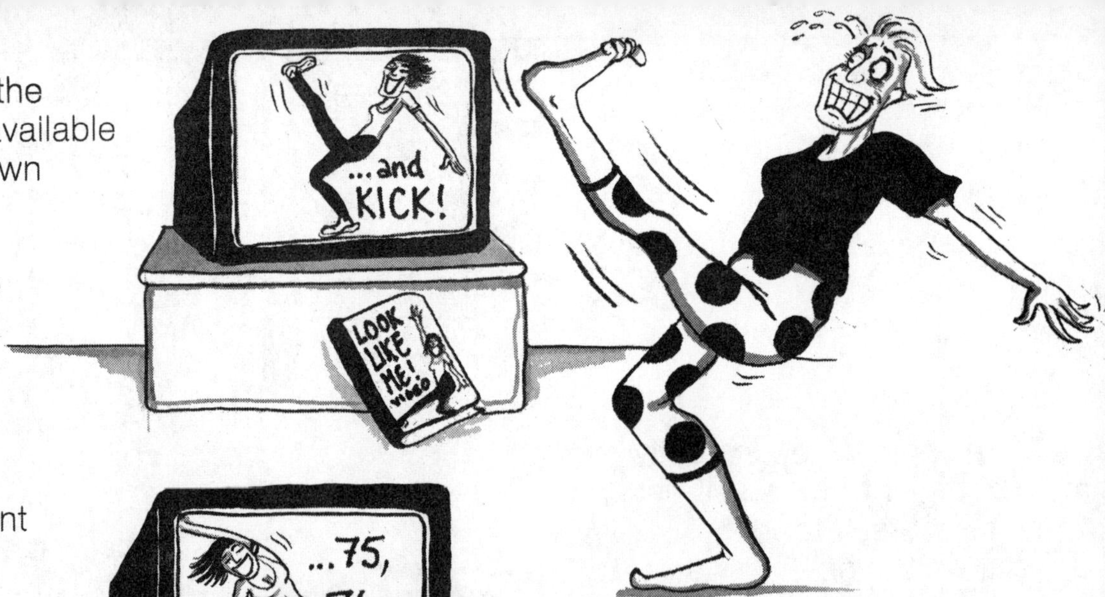
...and KICK!
LOOK LIKE ME! VIDEO

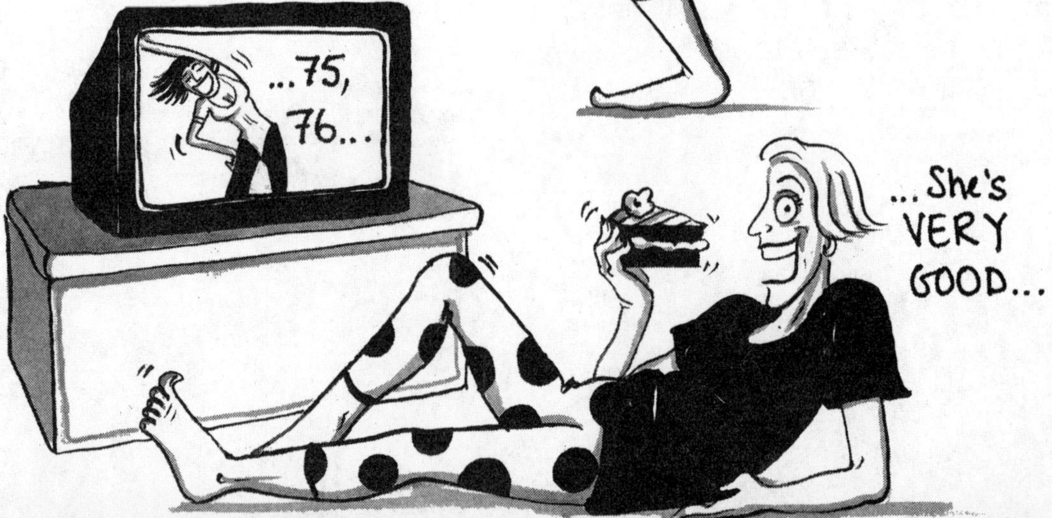
...75, 76...
...She's VERY GOOD...

You could whittle away your flab and thin out your savings by going to a HEALTH FARM.

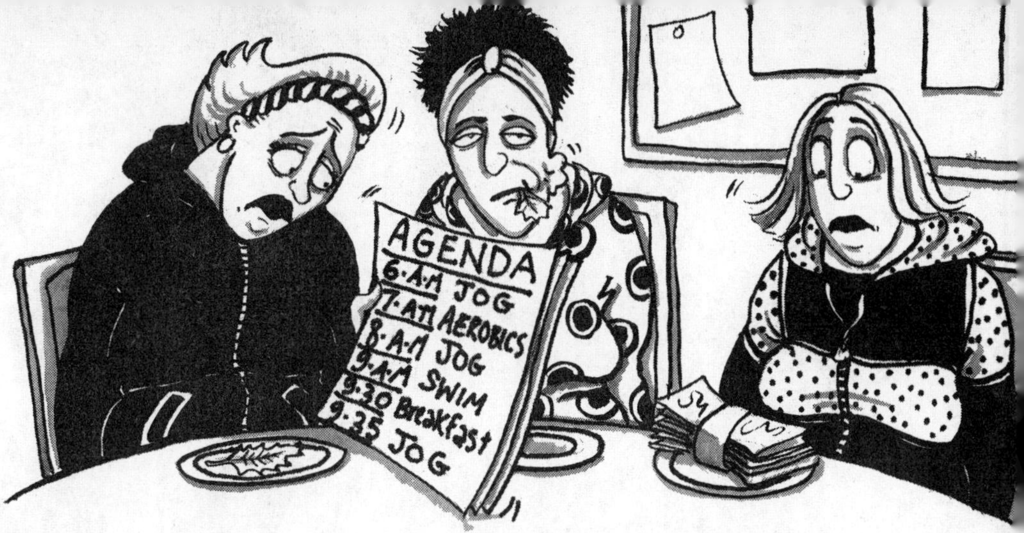
AGENDA
6.A.M JOG
7.A.M AEROBICS
8.A.M JOG
9.A.M SWIM
9.30 Breakfast
9.35 JOG

You could have a regular MASSAGE.

... Maybe you could try AEROBICS ...

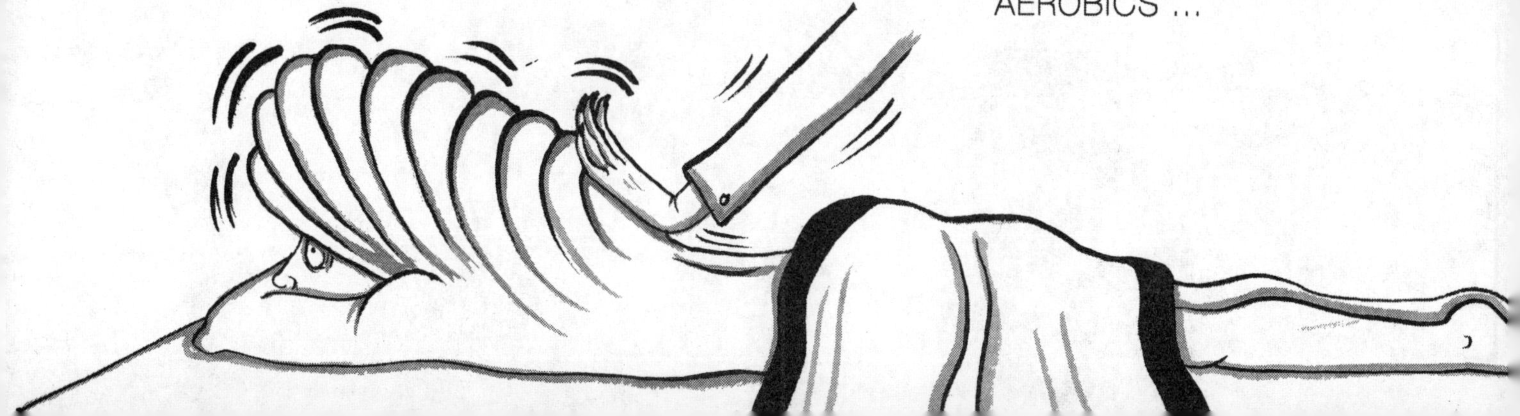

... or maybe NOT!

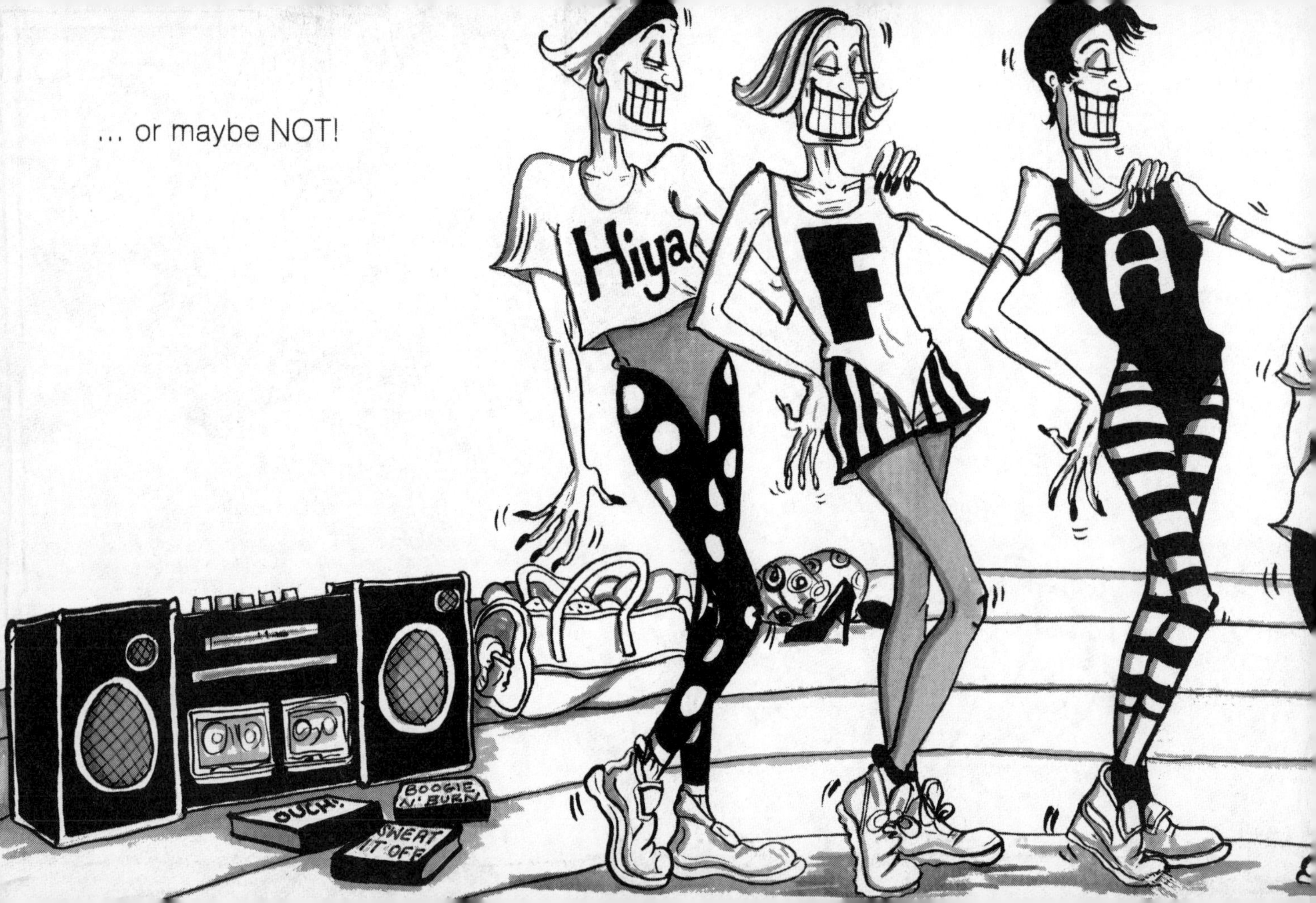

Hiya
F
A
OUCH!
BOOGIE N' BURN
SWEAT IT OFF

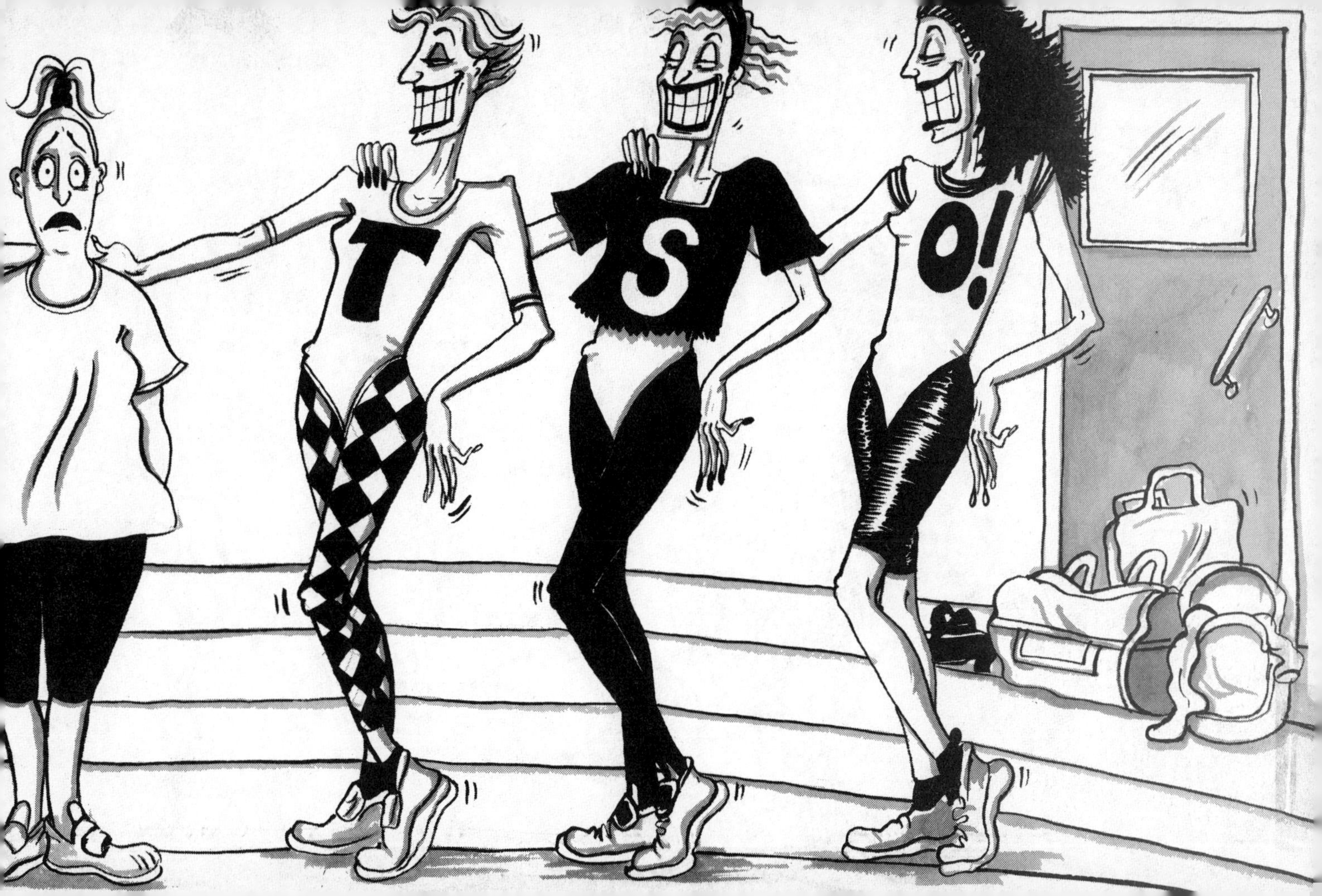
T
S
O!

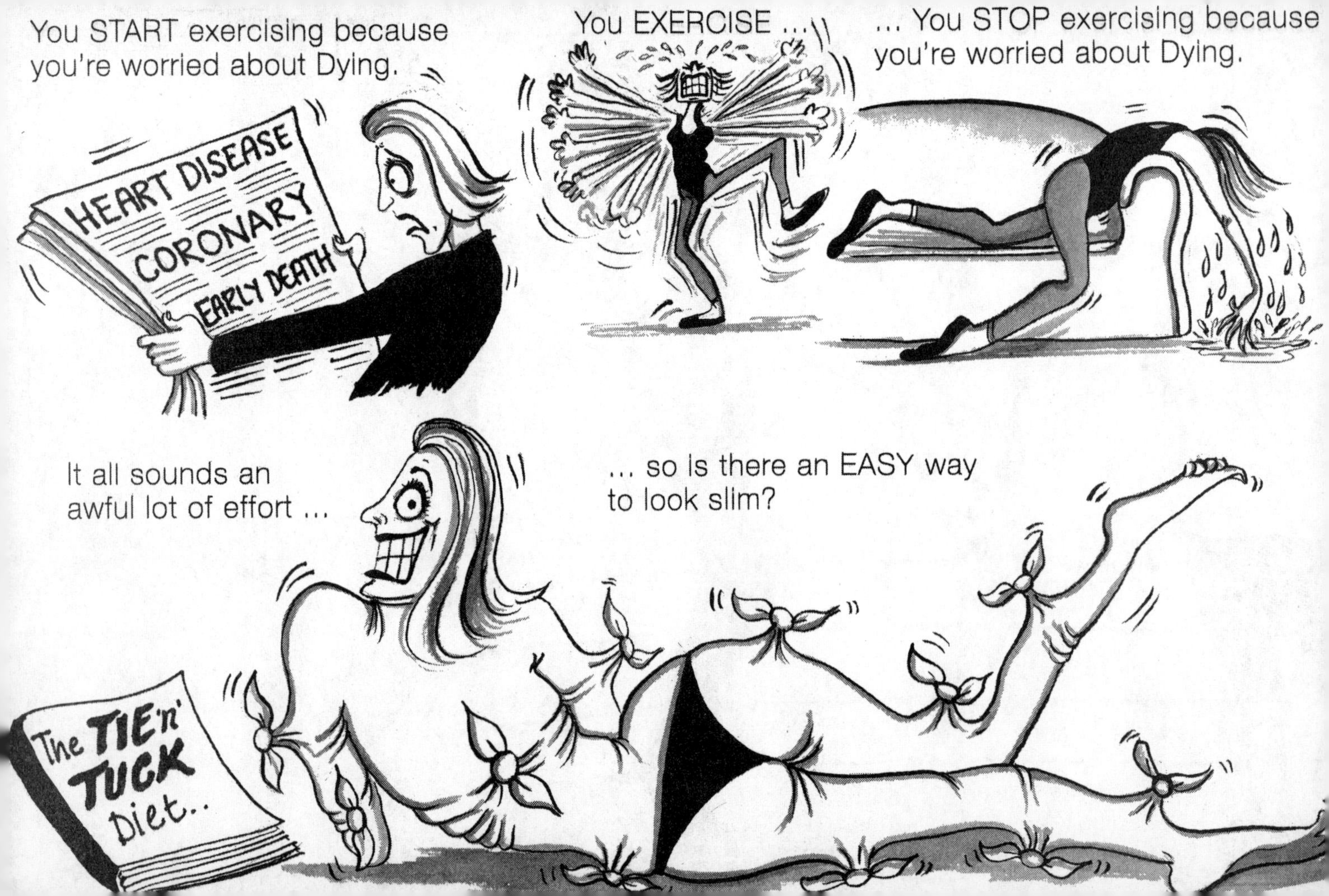
You START exercising because you're worried about Dying.
HEART DISEASE
CORONARY
EARLY DEATH
You EXERCISE ...
... You STOP exercising because you're worried about Dying.
It all sounds an awful lot of effort ...
... so is there an EASY way to look slim?
The TIE 'n' TUCK Diet..

PLASTIC SURGERY

Cut along dotted line...

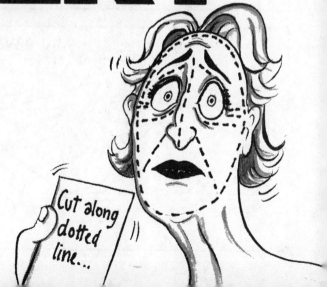

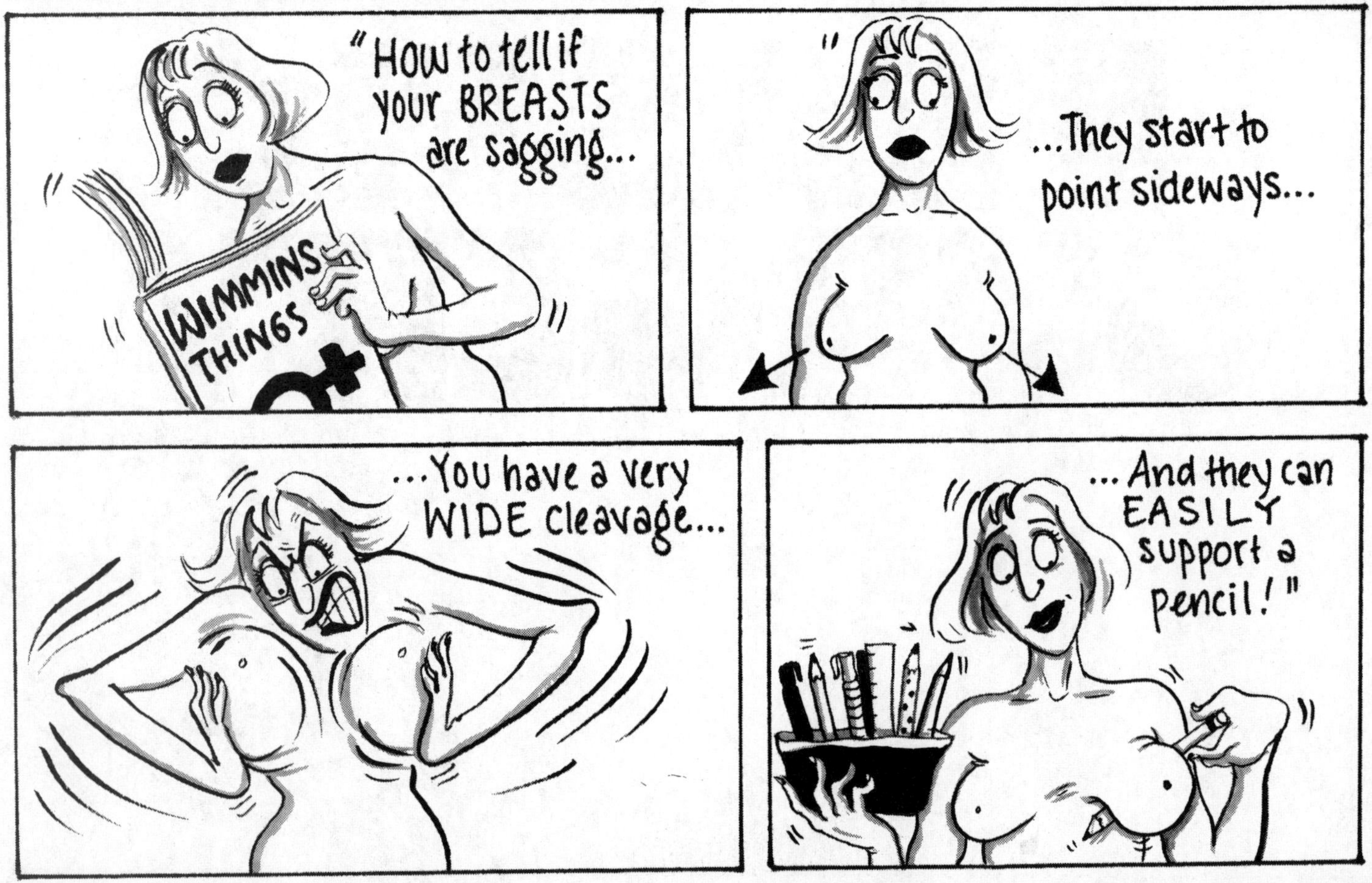
"HOW to tell if your BREASTS are sagging...
WIMMINS THINGS
...They start to point sideways...
...You have a very WIDE cleavage...
...And they can EASILY support a pencil!"

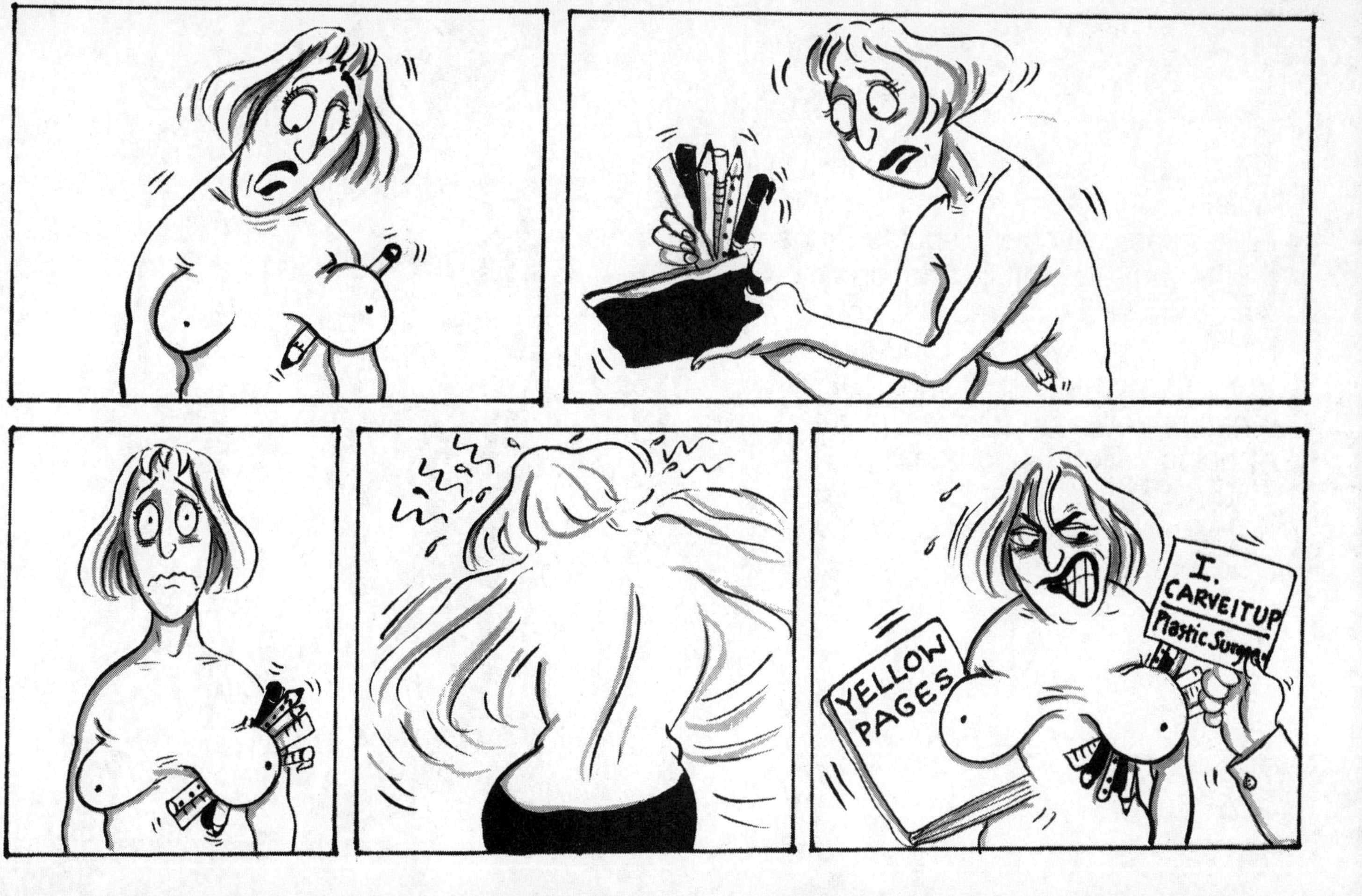
YELLOW PAGES
I. CARVEITUP
Plastic Surge

This has got to be the last resort. When you've held your stomach in for as long as you can; disguised those thighs with a carefully chosen wardrobe and you're STILL not happy ... then you're probably thinking about PLASTIC SURGERY. It can release you from a lifetime of being called Concorde or Thunderthighs: it can provide you with a new lease of life as well as a new profile ...

HIT LIST:
NOSE
BAGS
CHINS
NECK
BREASTS
UPPER
ARMS
LOWER
ARMS
STOMACH
WAIST
BOTTOM
INNER
THIGHS
OUTER
CALVES
BIG
TOE
EAR
LOBES

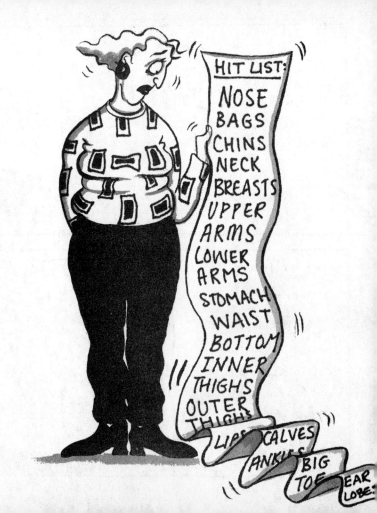

... but some women aren't satisfied with simple improvements and go for a complete reconstruction ...

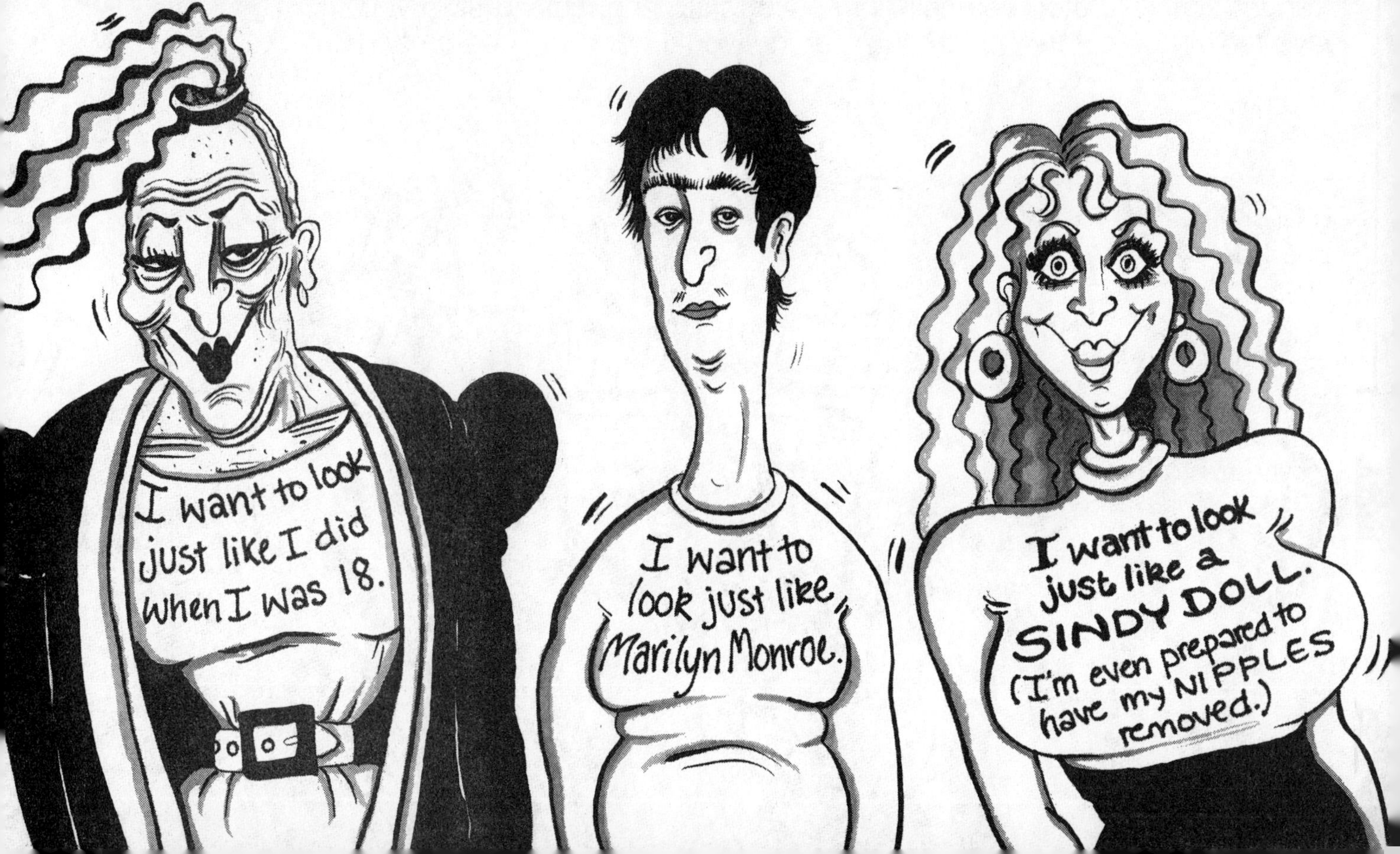

I want to look just like I did when I was 18.
I want to look just like Marilyn Monroe.
I want to look just like a SINDY DOLL. (I'm even prepared to have my NIPPLES removed.)

The CONSULTATION combines talking about your insecurities to a total stranger, trying to stop yourself from being sick, and making sure you leave feeling completely sure that your individual needs will be met.p103

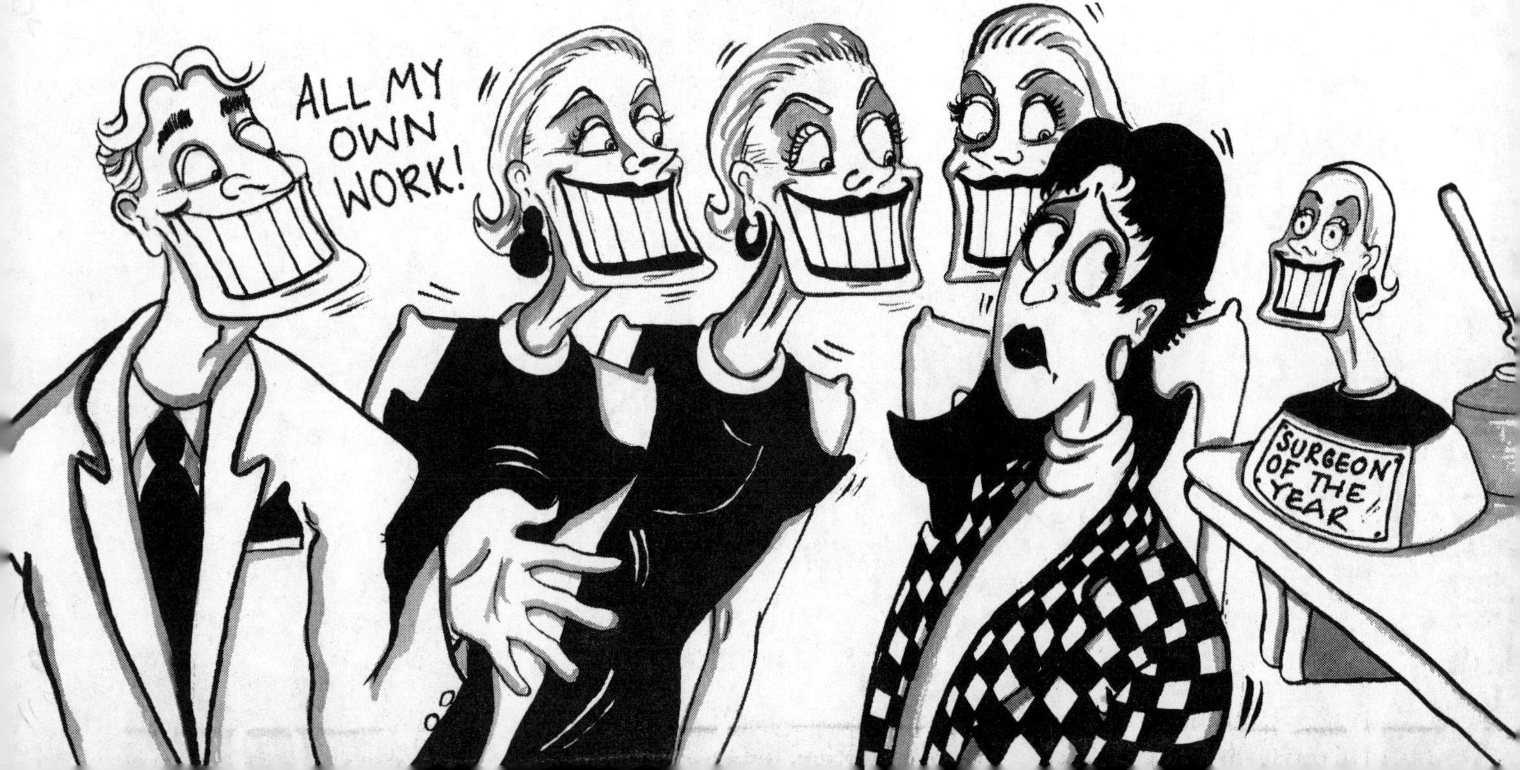
ALL MY OWN WORK!
SURGEON OF THE YEAR

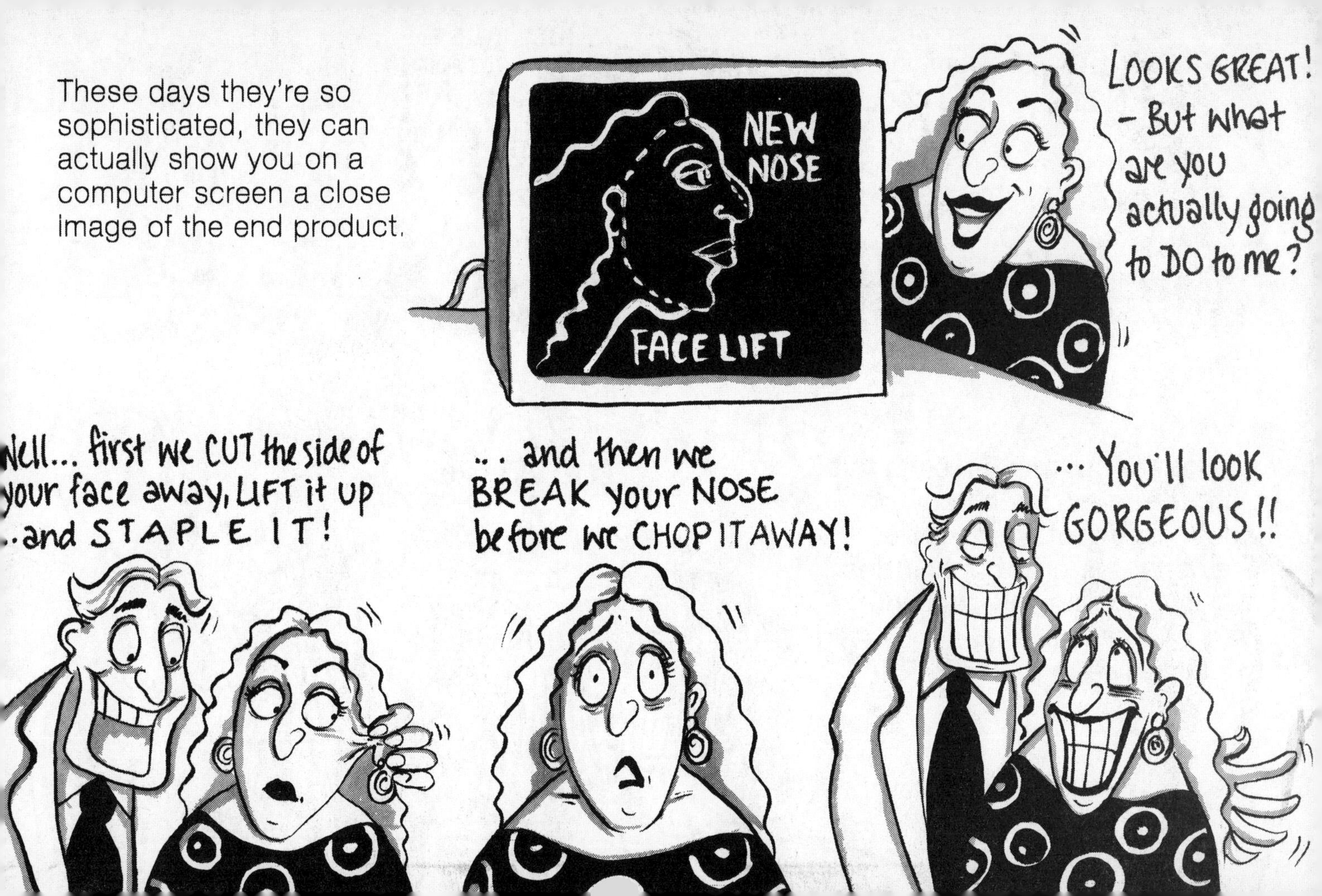
These days they're so sophisticated, they can actually show you on a computer screen a close image of the end product.
NEW NOSE
FACE LIFT
LOOKS GREAT! - But what are you actually going to DO to me?
Well... first we CUT the side of your face away, LIFT it up ..and STAPLE IT!
.. and then we BREAK your NOSE before we CHOP IT AWAY!
... You'll look GORGEOUS!!

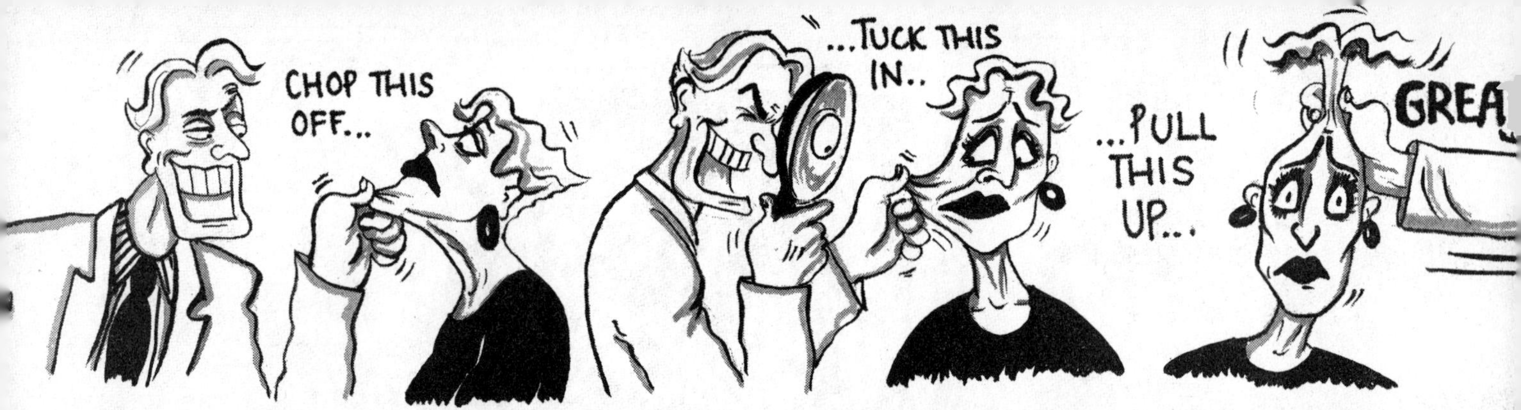
CHOP THIS OFF...
...TUCK THIS IN..
...PULL THIS UP...
GREA

The nature of the job means that plastic surgeons don't get too emotional about what they do. They spot the problem and deal with it in a practical, detatched manner. Imagine what it would be like to be MARRIED to one ...

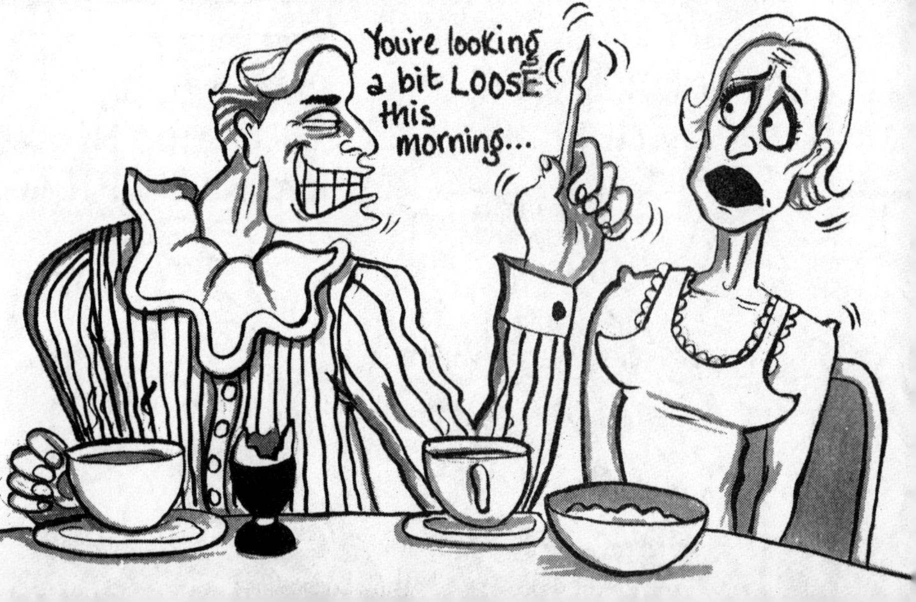
You're looking a bit LOOSE this morning...

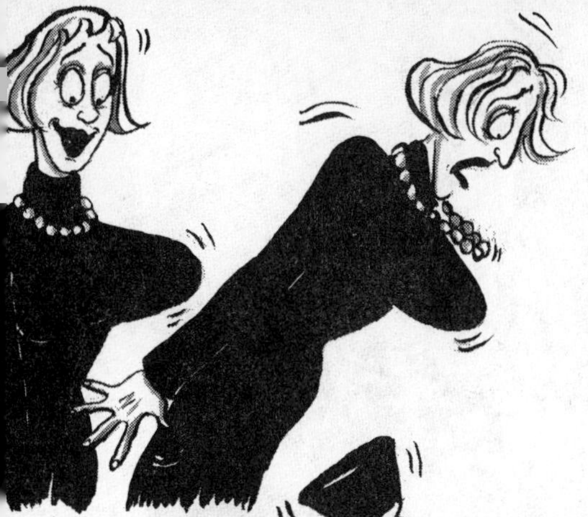

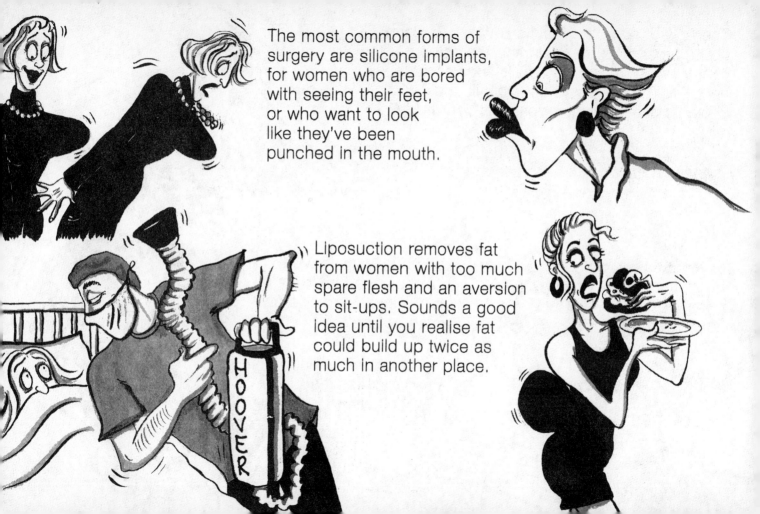

The most common forms of surgery are silicone implants, for women who are bored with seeing their feet, or who want to look like they've been punched in the mouth.

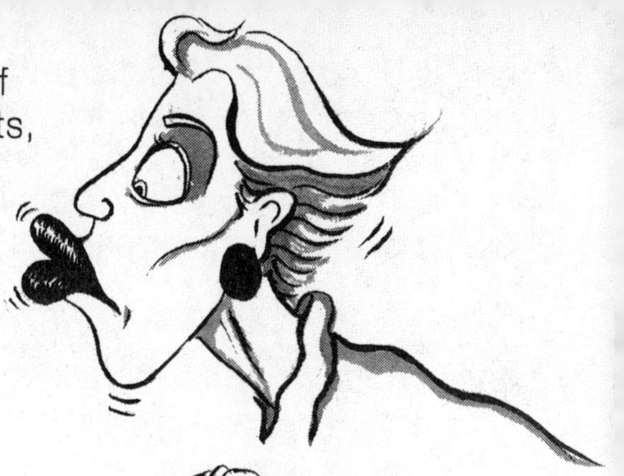

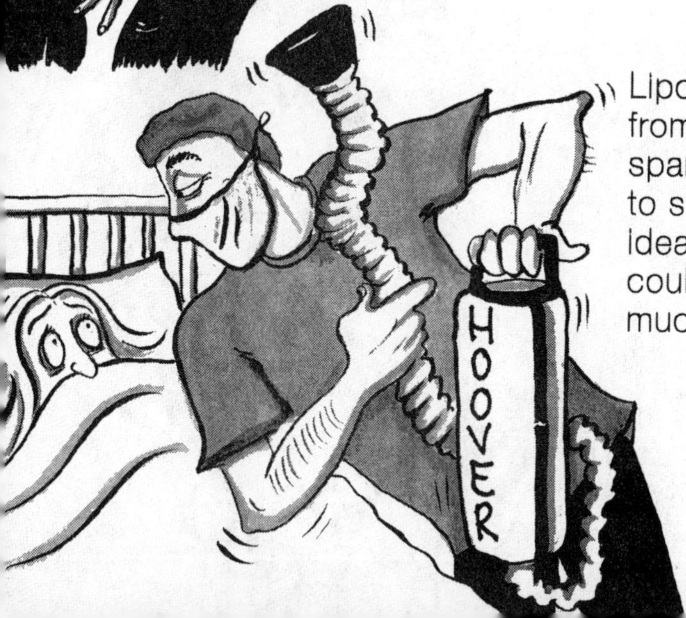
HOOVER

Liposuction removes fat from women with too much spare flesh and an aversion to sit-ups. Sounds a good idea until you realise fat could build up twice as much in another place.

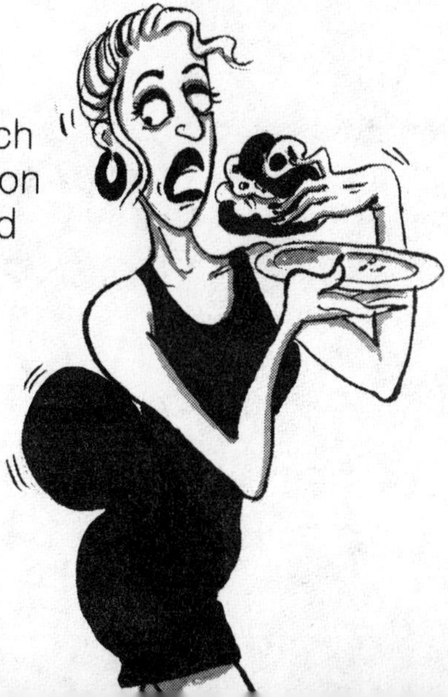

The only thing about Plastic Surgery to worry about (apart from the pain and the risk of mistakes) is that no-one really knows what happens after a few years. Do silicone implants seep into other parts of your body?

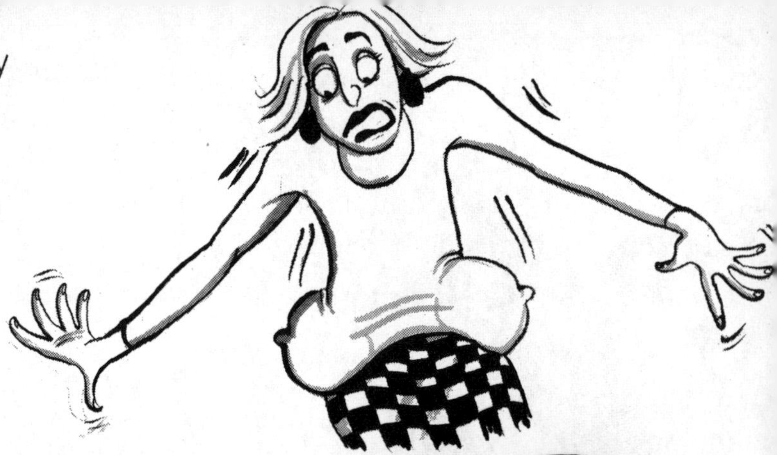

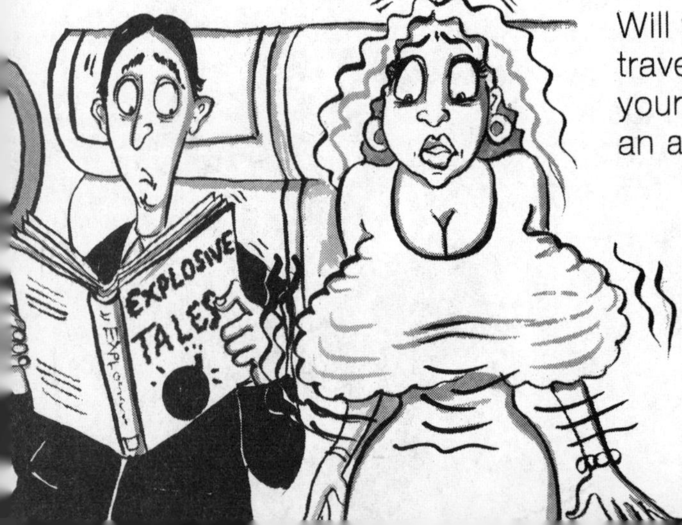
EXPLOSIVE
TALES

Will you always have to travel by sea just in case your breasts explode on an aeroplane?

... and what happens if your lips just don't wear down evenly?

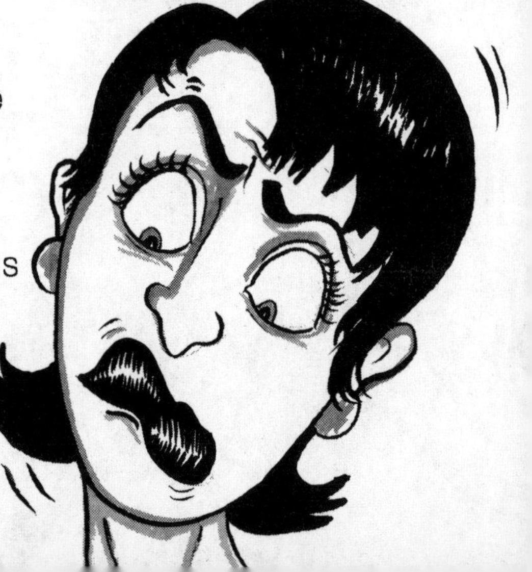

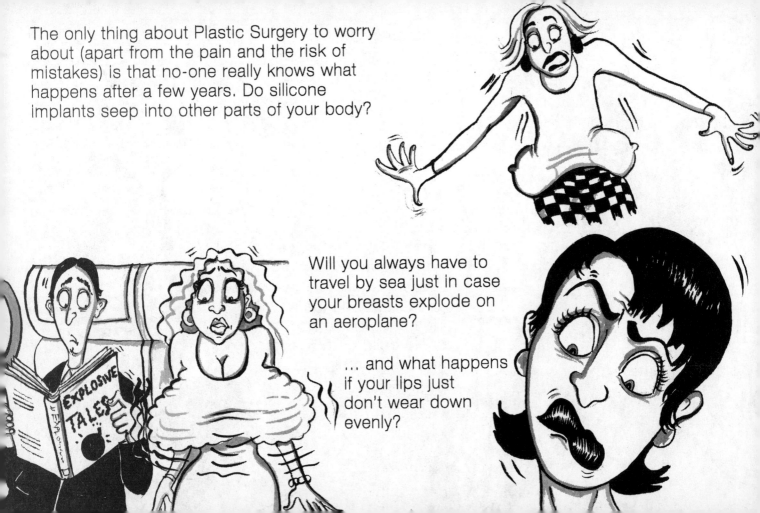

The best we can do is to keep a close eye on women who have had plastic surgery, so we can see exactly what effect it can have, before we even consider it. After all, you may have face lift after face lift to keep yourself looking young ... but how long have you got before your FACE COLLAPSES?

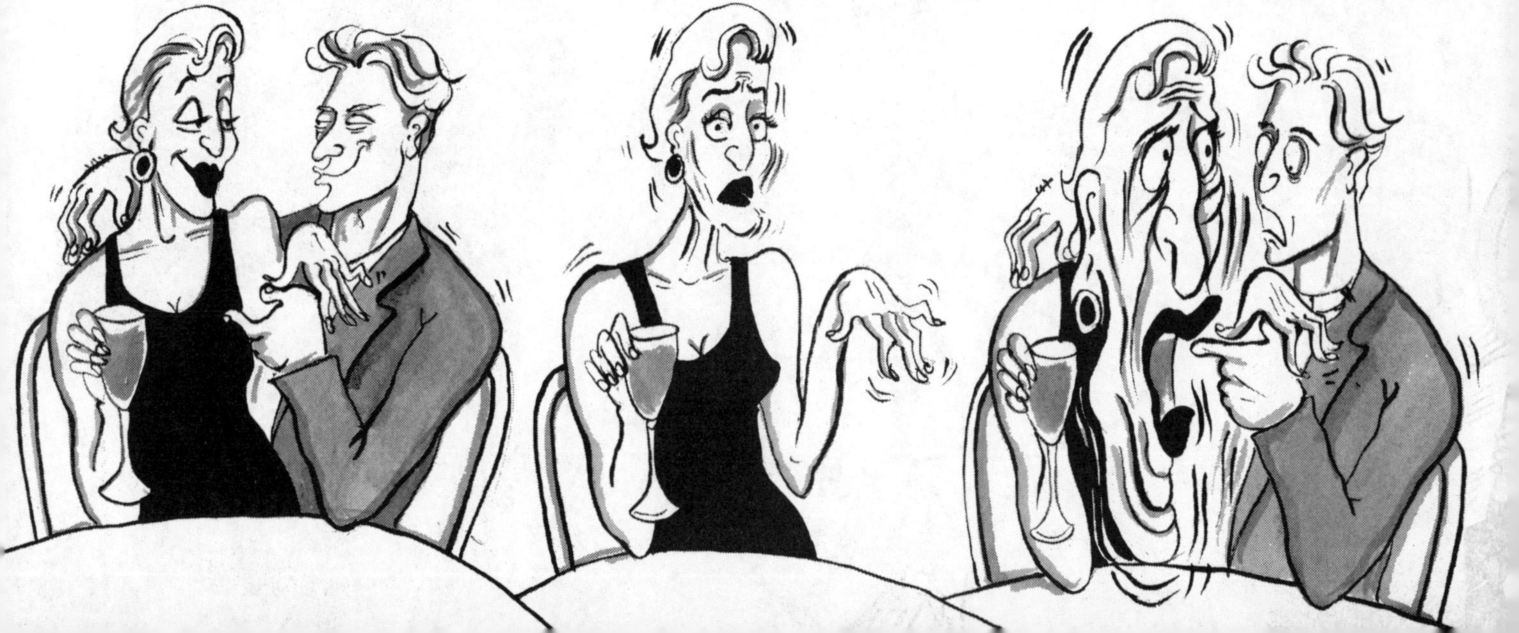

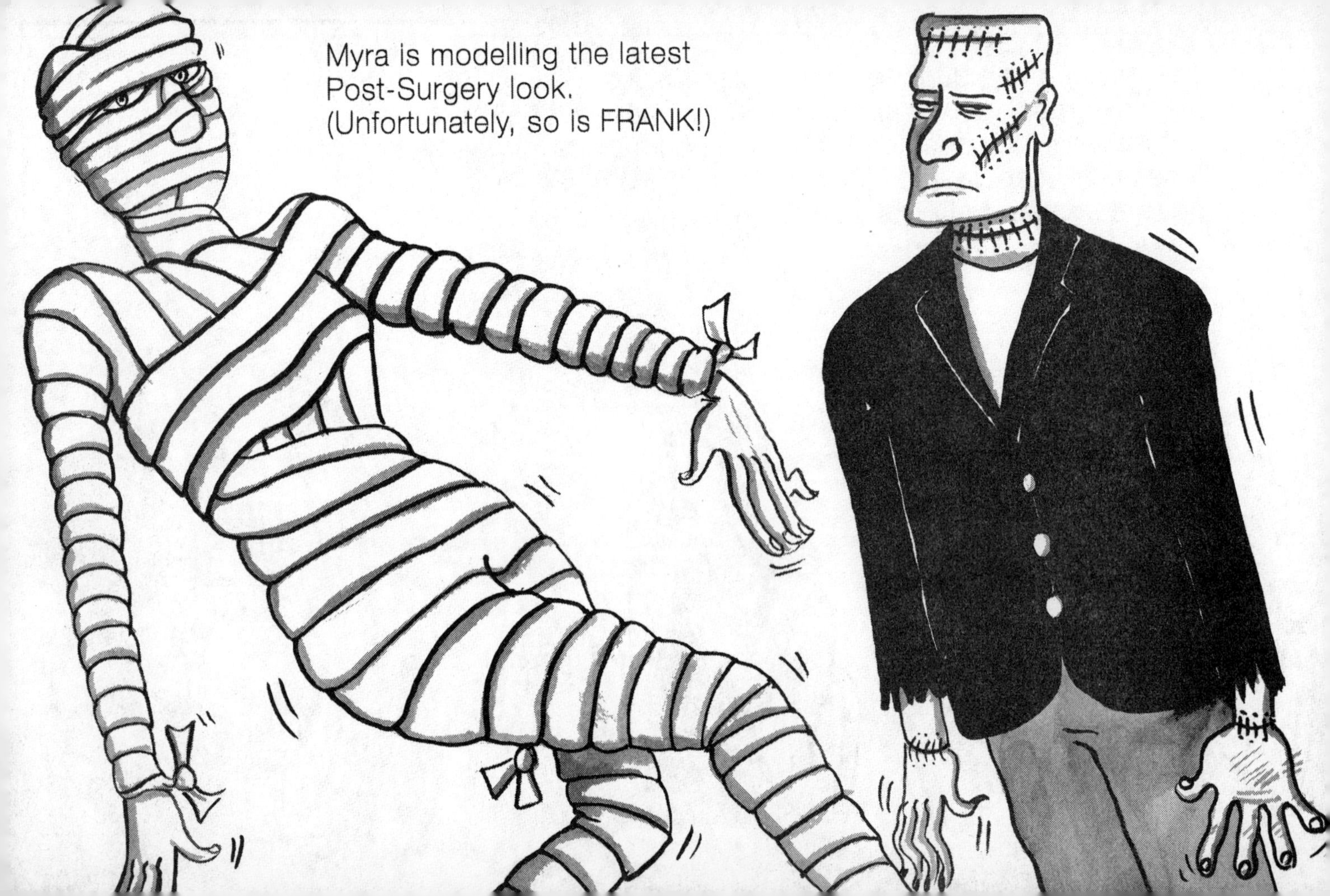
Myra is modelling the latest
Post-Surgery look.
(Unfortunately, so is FRANK!)

Unless crumpled faces and saggy bodies become desirable attributes, squeamish women like me will have no choice but to find pain-free alternatives to Plastic Surgery.

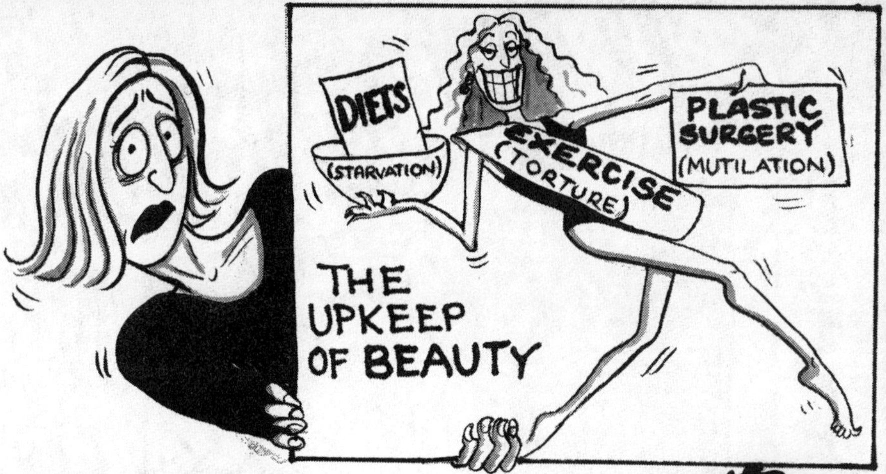
DIETS
(STARVATION)
EXERCISE
(TORTURE)
PLASTIC SURGERY
(MUTILATION)
THE UPKEEP OF BEAUTY

We could try looking SURPRISED for the rest of our lives ...

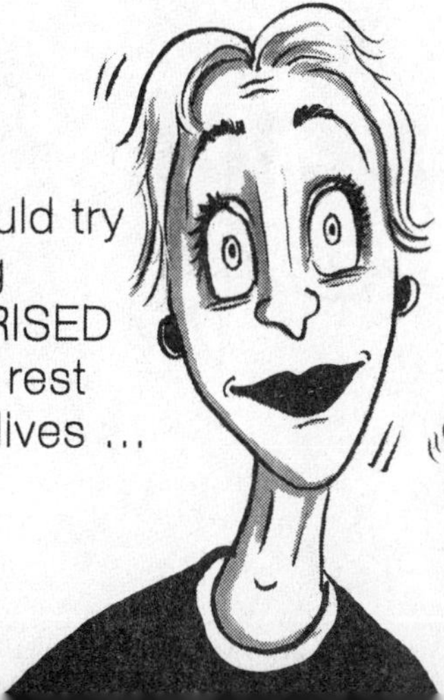

... surrounding ourselves with people who look a LOT older than us ...

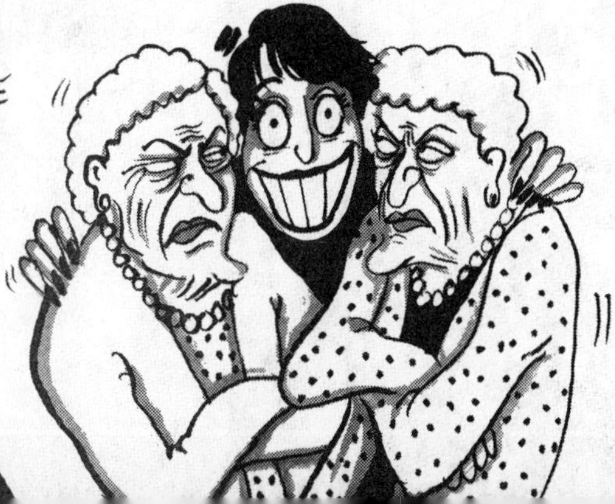

... or by wearing very TIGHT HEADBANDS!

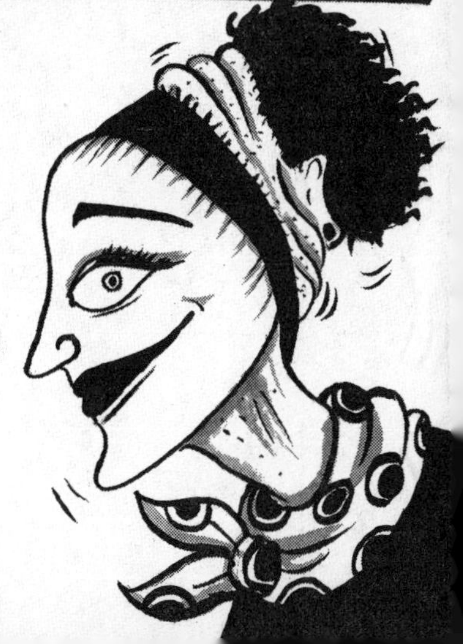

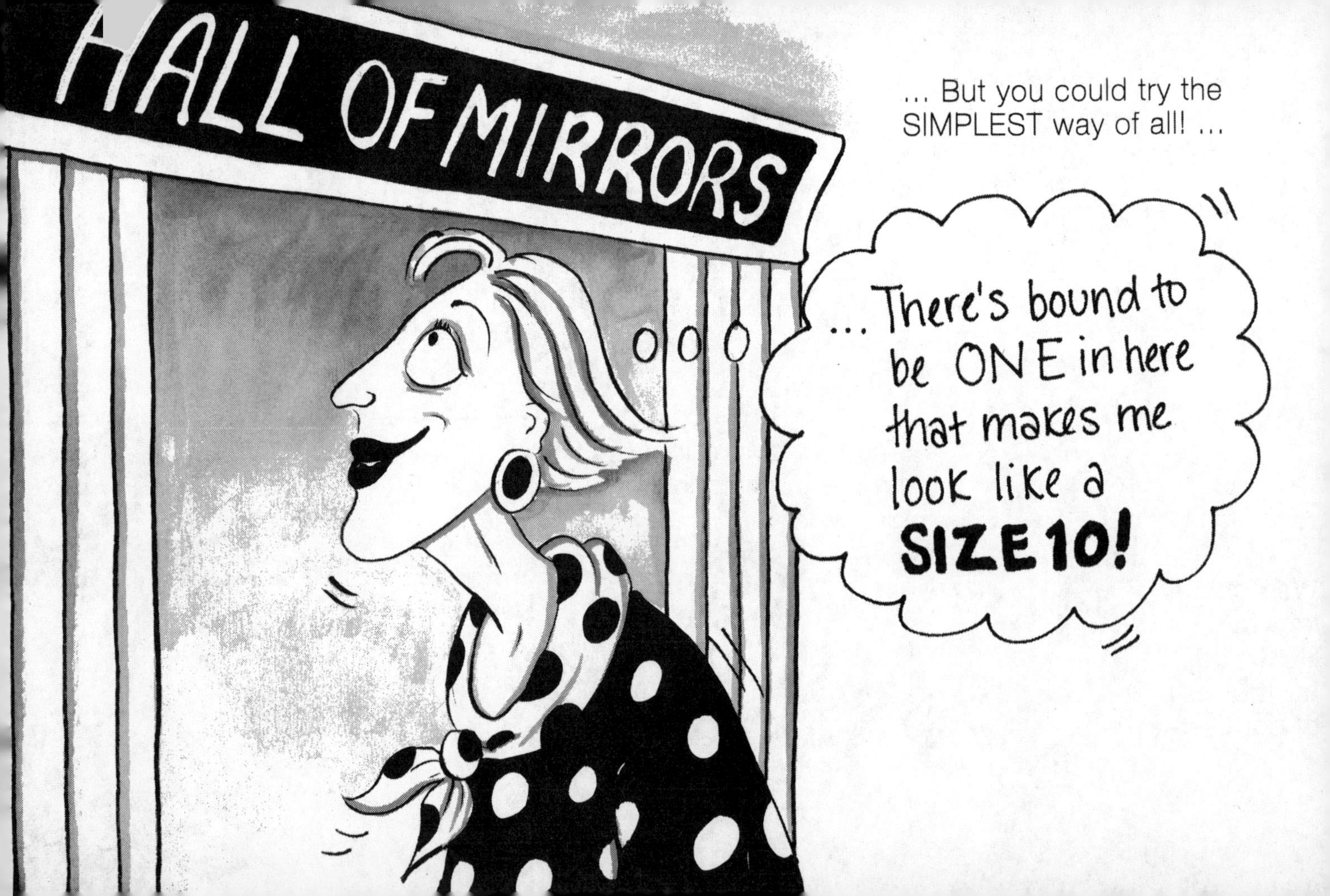
HALL OF MIRRORS
... But you could try the SIMPLEST way of all! ...
... There's bound to be ONE in here that makes me look like a SIZE 10!